Whitchurch Hospitals
Their History & Medical Care

Whitchurch Hospitals
Their History & Medical Care

by

John S. Clayton

Logaston Press

LOGASTON PRESS
Little Logaston, Logaston,
Woonton, Almeley, Herefordshire HR3 6QH

Published by Logaston Press 2004
Copyright text © John S. Clayton 2004

ISBN 1 904396 26 7

Printed in Great Britain by
Bell & Bain Ltd., Glasgow

Contents

Acknowledgments

I would like to thank the following: Mrs. Joan Barton and R.B. James, both well known local historians, Paul Anderton of Keele University, Mrs. Blower for information on Prees, the *Whitchurch Herald*, staff at the British Library, the Shropshire Research and Records Centre, the Wellcome Institute Library and Whitchurch Library, members of the Whitchurch History and Archaeology Group. Especially I would like to acknowledge secretarial help from a kind lady from my days in medical practice and, not least, my wife, who supported all my efforts and never failed to encourage me.

Introduction

I looked at the Rector's book in the glass case in St. Alkmund's Church, Whitchurch. It was open at the year 1794, and there was an account by the Rev. Francis Henry Egerton, Rector of Whitchurch and Myddle, in his own writing, of the building of a new House of Industry to replace the old Poor Law premises.

The Infirmary, which was detached from the House by a distance of 60ft., contained two wards for the sick; five beds for males and females and chambers for attendants.

The Cottage Hospital was built in 1886 on a site nearby. Both hospitals were administered separately until the start of the National Health Service in 1949 and they did became fully combined as the Community Hospital in 1990.

I wanted to know what medical care was really like for the ordinary citizen of Whitchurch over the ages. I worked through the centuries to my own lifetime and found eccentric and, I hope, interesting characters all the way.

I am not a trained historian, just a retired general practitioner, but with patience and a great deal of help from my friends, I found it rewarding. I trust you will do so too.

1 Early Medical Care

For at least four and a half million years human ancestors were hunters and gatherers, living in small groups comprising perhaps fifty members, and although they had a very tough life with many injuries, starvation and other problems, they had few 'illnesses'. They rarely stayed in one place for very long so there was no pollution or refuse problems and no domestic animals (a known source of disease).

About ten thousand years ago, at about the end of the last Ice Age, humans became farmers. They kept first of all dogs (with which to hunt), then horses and cattle and other livestock. Many began to live in permanent dwelling places and problems developed as they came in contact with rats, mice and lice.

In 3000 BC in the warm and fertile areas between Mesopotamia and Egypt, cities with populations as large as 50,000 were springing up. Many illnesses began to spread quickly from human to human and merchants, missionaries and marching armies rapidly spread infections.

In 1728–1686 BC the king of the dynasty of Babylon was Hammurabi. He was a powerful ruler who produced a code of medical behaviour which was recorded on a two-metre-high stele found in Iran in 1901 and now preserved in the Louvre. This gave specific instructions to the court physicians, its rules setting out even what they were to charge for treatment. These fees were based on a sliding scale, adjusting rewards as to whether the patient was a nobleman, commoner or slave. Awful fines for incompetence were recorded in Roy Porter's book *The Greatest Benefit to Mankind* in which he describes the penalties as follows:

> If a physician has performed a major operation on a lord with a bronze lancet and has saved the lord's life ... he shall receive ten shekels of silver (more than a craftsman's annual pay); but if he caused the death of such a notable, his hand would be chopped off. A doctor causing the death of a slave would have to replace him.

Medical care became important in these cities, and clay tablets from around 650 BC gave a description of many illnesses. In Nineveh, King Assurbanipal, who lived around 668–627 BC, had a library containing 30,000 clay tablets. Of these, at least 1,000 were concerned with medical matters and many illnesses were described.

The Babylonians saw the hand of god in everything. At that time there were seen to be three types of healers: a seer who went in for divination; a priest who conducted religious services and a physician who performed some simple surgical procedures, bandaging and the drugs employed. Certainly the Babylonian physician had a wonderful collection of preparations on which to draw. Some of their favourites were honey, mustard, senna and castor oil.

In Egypt, the Ebers papyrus of 1550 BC, the oldest surviving medical book, contains details of disease and the remedies, including spells and incantations, the use of garlic, helleborus and even opium and cannabis in the form of pills or ointments. Another papyrus discovered by Edwin Smith near Luxor is called *A Book of Wounds*. This describes how to reduce a dislocated jaw and to set other bones by the use of ox-bone splints. Other papyri deal with methods of detecting pregnancy and contraception, for which pulverized crocodile dung was mixed with honey. My source of information does not say how this was administered.

As in Mesopotamia the Egyptians had the same division of healers. One was Iri, Keeper of the Royal Rectum, presumably the pharaoh's enema expert. Enemas were widely used. We also hear of Imhotep 'he who comes in peace' who was chief vizier to Pharaoh Zozer. He designed pyramids and had a knowledge of astrology as well as being a physician. Under the pharaohs there was strong state control, and physicians were appointed to superintend public works, the army, burial grounds and the pharaoh's palace.

The Egyptians allowed mummification but the embalmers had a separate guild and were of low caste. They usually removed the brain through the nose by hooks but left the heart in place.

By 1000 BC Greece and its islands were growing in importance in terms of medical care. At first the influence of the gods was very significant and Asclepius the physician was regarded as the son of the god Apollo, sired of a mortal mother. It was his sign of two snakes entwined around a staff which is still regarded as the symbol of medicine. He was often shown accompanied by his three daughters: Hygeia, from whom comes the word hygiene, Panacea, from whom we have cure-all, and Aigle. Gods were still important when Homer in the *Iliad* asked for relief from the terrible plague of Athens

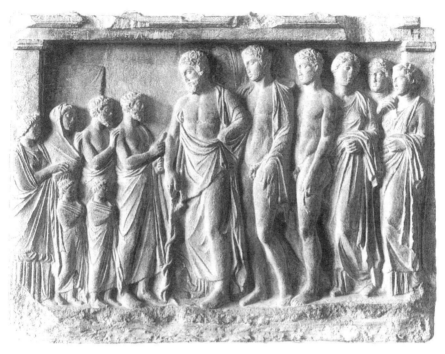

Votive relief to Asclepius, 350BC, who leans on his staff with its entwined snake. With him are his wife and sons, and daughters Hygeia, Aigle and Panacea, the former being the goddess of health

of 430–427 BC. Certainly the Greeks were very interested in keeping fit and record that they believed in exercise, gymnastics and diet. It was they, of course, who started the Olympic games in 776 BC.

By the third century BC most of the Greek islands had temples to Asclepius, where pilgrims used to go and stay overnight and hoped to receive visions during the night's 'temple sleep' and feel better from their illnesses in the morning.

The island of Cos was where Hippocrates was born. Hippocrates, 460–377 BC, did not believe that disease could be caused or even cured by supernatural forces such as gods, believing instead in careful physical examination. In his writings he set out his philosophy as follows: 'make frequent visits, always be especially careful with examinations, get to know the case more easily and you yourself will be more at ease'. He advised on diet and lifestyle, and as regards treatment it was important that this should, at the very least, do no harm to the patient. He also produced his famous theories about the humours—blood, yellow bile, black bile and phlegm—

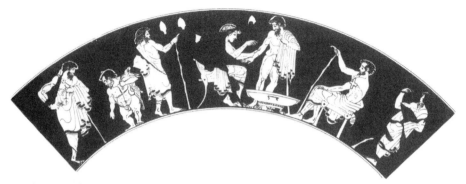

A scene from an Athenian doctor's surgery of the time of Hippocrates, painted around a perfume vase. In the centre the doctor treats a patient's arm, whilst others await their turn

and made many deductions regarding the best treatment and prognosis on that basis. He was very insistent on high standards of conduct, and set out the original Hippocratic Oath:

> I swear by Apollo the healer, by Aesculapius, by Health and all the powers of healing, and call to witness all the gods and goddesses that I may keep this Oath and Promise to the best of my ability and judgement.
>
> I will pay the same respect to my master in the Science as to my parents and share my life with him and pay all my debts to him. I will regard his sons as my brothers and teach them the Science, if they desire to learn it, without fee or contract. I will hand on precepts, lectures and all other learning to my sons, to those of my master and to those pupils duly apprenticed and sworn, and to none other.
>
> I will use my power to help the sick to the best of my ability and judgement; I will abstain from harming or wronging any man by it.
>
> I will not give a fatal draught to anyone if I am asked, nor will I suggest any such thing. Neither will I give a woman means to procure an abortion.
>
> I will be chaste and religious in my life and in my practice.
>
> I will not cut, even for the stone, but I will leave such procedures to the practitioners of that craft. Whenever I go into a house, I will go to help the sick and never with the intention of doing harm or injury. I will not abuse my position to indulge in sexual contacts with the bodies of women or of men, whether they be freemen or slaves.
>
> Whatever I see or hear, professionally or privately, which ought not to be divulged, I will keep secret and tell no one.

4

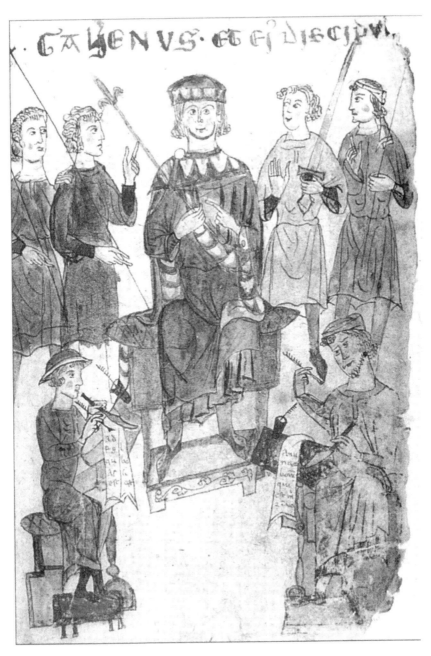

A 14th-century depiction of Galen surrounded by his pupils

> If, therefore, I observe this Oath and do not violate it, may I prosper both in my life and in my profession, earning good repute among all men for all time. If I transgress and forswear this Oath, may my lot be otherwise.

This was the oath sworn at a gathering of medical students in Sheffield where I qualified and is still sworn in many medical schools in America.

The Romans built on the basis of Greek medicine and many of their best doctors were Greeks. These included Soranus, who was interested particularly in problems of childbirth; Agnodice, an Athenian lady, who, according to legend, was so distressed by the anguish of women who would rather die than be examined by a man, that she studied and practised medicine; and Dioscorides, a Greek surgeon in Nero's army who wrote several books on herbal remedies. Outstanding amongst them was Galen who was born in Pergamon, Turkey, in 129 AD. In Rome he was appointed physician to the gladiators, a job which helped both his anatomical knowledge and surgical skill. He also became a very close friend of the emperors, particularly of Emperor Marcus Aurelius, who was his patient. Galen absorbed all the Hippocratic Corpus teachings adding a few others like venesection (letting blood from the veins) to cool the body. These views dominated medicine for well over the next thousand years, medical knowledge changing very little until Harvey and Galileo began to challenge what had become the *status quo*.

2 Medicine in Britain

At Whixall Moss (a world scientific site) in north Shropshire there is evidence of some kind of settlement in the finding of two bodies in the bog. It is thought that one of these, found in 1889 a mile from the Waggoners Inn, might be that of a Bronze Age man. Techniques of analysis were not, of course, available in those days, but from the depth at which the body was found and from pollen, the remains of trees around and other analyses, it is suggested that he lived some time between 3,000 and 2,000 BC. The discovery was related in the *Whitchurch Herald* and *Nantwich Chronicle* who stated that two men cutting peat found the body in their second and third layers, at a depth of 5 feet. He was lying flat out at full length, face downwards. The District Coroner was informed and the body was subsequently reburied in Whixall churchyard. This was the first Whitchurch citizen of whom we have any knowledge.

When the Romans arrived in Britain under Julius Caesar in 54 BC they found the island inhabited by what was described by Tacitus as 'warlike tribes'. In AD 43–47 the Emperor Claudius invaded Britain in force and advanced to the Midlands, in due course arriving in the territory of a tribe that the Romans called the Cornovii, whose lands lay in the Cheshire and North Shropshire plains.

It is not known how much resistance the Cornovii made but the legions soon set up two bases in their territory: Wroxeter (*Viroconium*) which was built by the XIIII Legion, and Chester, the base of the XX Legion before it was moved, in part, to construct Hadrian's Wall in 122–127 AD. *Mediolanum*—the place on the mid plain—now Whitchurch, started as a sort of 'Bed and breakfast station' supplying the legions on the roads from London to Chester and Wroxeter to Chester.

The Roman army set aside special buildings (*valetudinaria*) for the treatment of their sick and wounded, including their domestic slaves. Their military hospitals were built to a standard plan with individual cells off a long corridor, a large top-lit hall, latrines and baths. There is an example of this in Inchtuthill in Scotland and there is evidence that there was a similar building in Chester.

In fortified towns like Chester the Romans had a sophisticated system of water supply, collecting clean water from reservoirs and keeping their drinking water well away from the drainage sewers to prevent disease. Underfloor heating using a system of hypocausts was another ingenious invention of the Romans. They had hot and cold baths and their use was a social occasion. This standard of hygiene was never achieved in Britain again until the 19th century, after Queen Victoria's consort, Prince Albert, died of typhoid.

Areas called the *canabae* contained shops and taverns, and there were areas for sex and recreation, and the public baths. Chester also had an amphitheatre, half of which is still visible today. It was excavated in the 1960s and is the largest stone-built example in Britain, with tiers of seats which might have held up to 7,000 spectators.

As regards medical care, the Romans used surgical instruments, which again were not dissimilar from those of the 19th century. There were knives and scalpels for making incisions, spatulas for mixing medicines, and a wide range of ointments were used as a poultice with herbs of thyme and garlic. There were eye specialists similar to our present day oculists, prescribing their own remedies for eye conditions. In addition, offerings were made to their gods, many of them incorporated from the Greek pantheon, to ward off evil spirits.

Roman *Mediolanum* was investigated by the archaeologist G.D.B. Jones in 1965–66, and was found to contain, besides the original fortifications, a Flavian fort from 75–100 AD. There was also a building thought to date from the mid 2nd or early 3rd century. It was here that was found an adult male skeleton, alongside which were fragments of pottery, pointing to the death occurring in the first quarter of the 4th century. The skeleton was of a young man, probably aged between 20 and 30 years. The cause of his death, as given by Dr. J. Gask, might have been due to trephining, the incision perhaps made by an instrument similar in effect to the present day circular saw with its projecting spike. A disc of bone 27mm. in diameter had been removed from the right lobe of the skull. Trephining has actually been carried out from prehistoric times, possibly for injuries or severe pains in the head, perhaps even for a painful wisdom tooth or to let out evil spirits. (Excavations in Anglo-Saxon cemeteries have revealed skulls which had suffered trephining).

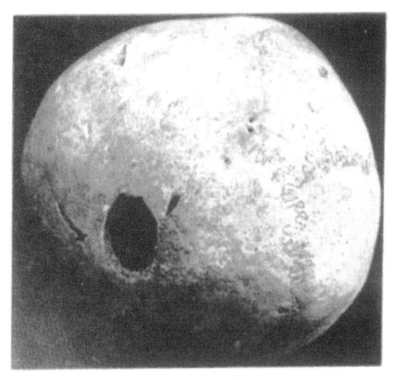

Trephined skull from Mediolanum

In AD 313 the Roman Emperor Constantine gave official recognition to Christianity. As Christian monasteries were set up in Britain they became real economic centres providing help in their own communities. in those days the medical care they offered simply meant rest, food, herbs, the binding of wounds and a safe haven (which only churches could provide).

Luke, one of the original disciples, known as 'The Beloved Physician', gave his instructions for caring for the sick and needy, a role soon adopted by Christian churches. In 390 AD, Fabiola, a wealthy Roman lady, converted to Christianity and devoted her life to caring for the sick in Rome, the first person reported as following this route.

The Venerable Bede, 672–735, lived his life in a monastery in Jarrow in Northumbria and made a significant advance in medical care since he possessed many medical writings which he was able to translate for the first time into English.

There was also the use of leeches and blood letting. A 10th-century document called the *Leechbook* describes these procedures and a wide range of herbal cures. Latin recipes were simplified by removing the more exotic ingredients and interweaving local remedies. Many diseases were also 'cured' by prayers and by invoking saints' names.

Wenlock Priory provides a good example of medical care in Shropshire. It was first established in AD 680, catering for both men and women. After 1040, it became a settlement for monks from the Abbey of Cluny in France. It contains a 12th-century infirmary, a single-storey building where sick, old or infirm monks and lay brothers were housed. A second storey was added at a later date to provide a warming room, dormitory and reredorter (toilet block). The infirmary had its own chapel, kitchen and cloister. Before entering the refrectory the monks washed in the lavatorium, an octagonal building with open arcades which supported a roof, where sixteen monks could wash simultaneously. The trough had plugholes for drainage, and is supported by a circular base around which were several elaborately carved panels depicting Christ and the apostles. Two of these panels survive. Such a building is rare in the country but common on the Continent.

The barber surgeons used to perform minor operations on the kitchen table and heroic surgery and amputations in ships' cabins in war time. A group of surgeons, whose duty was clearly to treat the wounds of the troops, accompanied Henry V's Agincourt campaign in 1415. Notable medieval surgeons included Guy de Chauliac in Paris and John of Arderne who, in the 15th century, was an expert on anal fistulas and deep abscesses in that region, thought to be particularly prevalent in members of the knightly class who spent a lot of time on horseback in heavy armour. Surgeons still did the same operations as the Romans. Using almost identical instruments they were able to trephine skulls, treat nasal polyps, cataracts, bladder stones, fractures and dislocations and injuries from arrows, and other wounds requiring suture. It was not until 1840 that anaesthesia and antiseptics made surgery a better proposition.

Lord John Talbot, perhaps Whitchurch's most famous citizen, was born at Blakemere in 1386. The accounts of the Talbot household for the years 1394–1425 make fascinating reading. Made in Latin by the house steward or seneschal, they include an entry for 'necessities' which included a medicine called Colikapassyon for Lord Furnival (John Talbot's step-father). More attention, however, is given to the rituals of burial. When Ankaret, a member of the family, died aged five years, money was given to the minstrels, and her mother sent a gentlewoman to Holywell on a pilgrimage.

In 1545, John Gerard was born in the nearby town of Nantwich in Cheshire. He started his career as a plantsman and had his own garden in Holborn, publishing a catalogue of its contents in 1596. This listed more than one thousand species—'the first professedly complete catalogue ever published of the contents of a single garden', in the words of the botanist Agnes Arber. (The list includes the first reference to potatoes being grown in England). Gerard was also very interested in growing herbs for medical purposes, and his *The Herball or Generall Historie of Plants* was the most complete herbal then published in English, not just translated from an overseas text. Amongst his friends were many botanists and also Sir Walter Raleigh.

John Gerard also provided an enthralling picture of the state of medicine in his time, not only of preferred remedies, but even of the doctors' attitudes. How, for example (with what length of tongue concealed in cheek), does one read this:

> The roote of Salomons Seale stamped while it is fresh and greene, and applied, taketh away in one night or two at the most, any bruse, black or blew spots, gotten by fats or womens wilfulness, in stumbling upon their hastie husbands fists, or such like.

He is known to have accompanied the Lord Mayor of London, Sir John Wolstenholme, of the London Virginia Company, while he was surveying the laying of London's water supply. He rose eventually to become Master of the Barber Surgeons Company in 1607. Incidentally, another contemporary of Gerard was Sir John Harrington, who in 1596 was credited as being the first man to invent the water closet toilet.

In England the numbers of hospitals and almshouses totalled almost five hundred by 1400, though few were of any size or significance.

In 1536 Henry VIII, for reasons of his own, 'stripped' all the churches and especially the medieval monasteries, and in doing this greatly reduced the capacity for medical care. After the Reformation only three main hospitals in London survived: St. Batholomew's; St. Thomas's—which had a master, six brethren and three lay sisters to look after forty people; and Bethlem which was founded in the 14th century for 'distracted people', a hospital for the insane. Just outside London, in St. Giles-in-the-Fields, there was a hospital for lepers, called a lazaretto. Another hospital was St. Leonard's of York which had two hundred and twenty-five sick and poor in 1287.

Stuart Times

Great advances were made in scientific understanding during the 17th century. The century opened with the time of Galileo, both scientist and mathematician, and continued with Isaac Newton, who was born in 1642 the year that Galileo died—in the middle of the English Civil War. There were many others. William Harvey, the son of a yeoman farmer, graduated from Cambridge in 1597, practised in London and studied under Fabrio at the University of Padua in Northern Italy. In 1628 he wrote *De Notu Cordis*—'The Heart is a Pump', the theory of blood circulation, which he dedicated to King Charles I.

However, the discoveries that were made did not permeate down into clinical practice until, in some cases, even the 19th century. During the Stuart era most doctors from the College of Physicians were clustered around the Court in London, and continued spouting the ideas of the ancient Greeks regarding the four humours. The possible exception was Thomas Sydenham who was greatly admired in England as the English Hippocrates.

Sydenham had served as captain of horse in the Parliamentarian army during the Civil War. In 1647 he went to Oxford and in 1655 began practising in London. Over his life he wrote many books, mostly in Latin, but also in English, as in the first chapter of *The Collection of Acute Diseases including Smallpox and Measles*, published by Henry Bonwicke in 1687. According to the publisher this small book was very useful for men who attend the army or go to sea. In his chapter Dr. Sydenham records the course of an illness and the value of 'Eyesight Observation' just as Hippocrates did. His treatment for smallpox and measles was as follows: The patient should stay in bed until the sixth day, should not need more clothes to wear or a fire in his chamber but only open air. He could drink freely of small beer, milk and water and eat oatmeal and apples but he was forbidden wine and flesh. He made no recommendations for blood letting, purges or clysters (enemas), all of which were very popular in the 17th and indeed 18th centuries.

In several cases he recommended Diacodium, a concoction of 24 heads of white poppy, well dried, in 8 pints of fountain water. He also used liquid Laudanum (Morphine): 'Thomas Millington, a fellow collegiate and a good friend joyn'd with me in treating my son William Sydenham who recovered from measles in 1670'.

He became a member of the Royal College of Physicians in 1676 and died in 1689. His teachings were followed in the next century by further practitioners, including one from Chester, John Haygarth, who was interested particularly in epidemics of smallpox and typhus.

Over the rest of England there were also some university trained doctors. Many surgeon/apothecaries were not academically trained but were good at minor surgery and the compounding of herbs, their learning being handed down often from father to son. Their limited resources were notably stretched at times of plague.

The Plague

The plague was a terrible medical problem causing much tragedy and suffering, starting from the first recorded outbreak which affected the Roman Empire — the Antonine Plague of AD 165. The Black Death reached its peak in 1348 when twenty million inhabitants of Europe, possibly a quarter of the population, perished. It remained active in Europe up until 1800, when it still persisted in the Far East and the Americas. The causal organism was a flea whose host was the black rat. It reached humans when the rat died and the flea searched for another host and found a human. The microbe itself was not finally identified until 1894 by the French bacteriologist Alexandre Yersin of the Pasteur Institute — so it is now called *Yersinia pestis.*

One of the many outbreaks of the plague in England was in 1563, when a quarter of London's population died. It was laid down by the Privy Council that parish clerks would have to make weekly returns of plague deaths. These were called Bills of Mortality and to prepare them each parish was expected to appoint a 'searcher', usually a local elderly lady, to make the diagnosis.

There were further outbreaks of the plague in 1578 and 1582. An epidemic in 1593 carried off 18,000 people in the City of London alone. The plague greeted James I's accession in 1603 by massacring 30,000 and when Charles I came to the throne in 1625 another 40,000 died.

Shrewsbury was affected by plague in 1650 and later that year the plague hit Whitchurch from August through to January 1651. Research by J.F.D. Shrewsbury into the plague in Whitchurch showed the annual burials for the year 1645–55 and the monthly burials for the years 1648, 1649 and 1650. The information on the graph overleaf clearly shows the plague cases beginning in August 1650 and running through into January 1651.

An even worse outbreak of the plague occurred in London from June to December 1665. In his *Diary* Pepys gives a glimpse of how it was possible to keep a normal life going with the plague around him. He sent his wife to live in Woolwich where he was working as secretary to the Naval Board, whilst he commuted to and from the City by river. He kept a close eye on the mortality figures and describes how the bells tolled at the churches. In

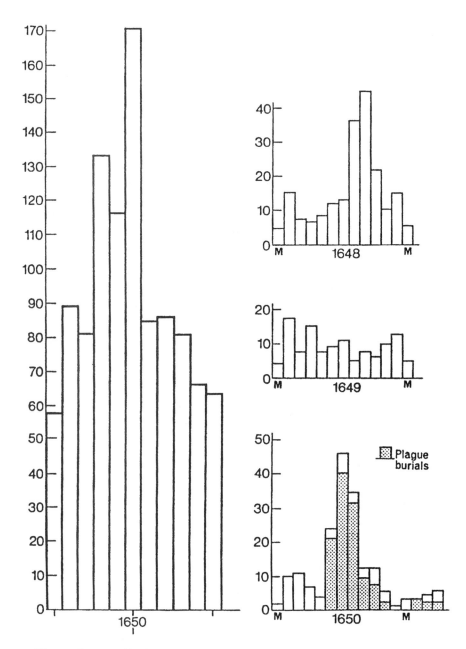

The epidemic of bubonic plague in Whitchurch in 1650, showing annual burials for the years 1645–55 and monthly burials for the years 1648, 1649, and 1650–1

some parts of the city it was necessary to bury the dead even in daylight because the nights were not sufficiently long. He was worried about his good friend and neighbour, Dr. Burnett of Fanchurch Street, and later in the *Diary* he says that he passed his house and saw that he had caused himself to be shut up of his own accord. Records show that after attending many cases Dr. Burnett died.

In June 1665 Pepys described a heatwave—'The hottest day that ever I felt in my life'. He saw red crosses springing up on houses in Drury Lane with the message 'Lord have mercy upon us'. People began to leave the town, particularly the wealthy. Clergymen abandoned their flocks, doctors fled their patients and in July the King, court and judges joined the stampede (the next six months were uniquely execution free). The Lord Mayor was one who remained. There was a rigidly enforced quarantine. JPs set up pesthouses in Marylebone, Soho Fields and Stepney and the Lord Mayor ordered the eradication of all dogs and cats, in the belief that they spread pestilence. Pepys reckoned that 40,000 dogs and perhaps five times as many cats were killed as part of a perfect recipe for safeguarding the rats!

Another who wrote about the plague was Daniel Defoe. In his *A Journal of the Plague Year* written in 1722, Defoe describes a Bill of Mortality for London in September 1665 which gave the following causes of death:

> Abortive 5, Aged 43, Ague 2, Apoplexies and Suddenly 2, Bleeding 2, Burnt in his bed at St. Giles Cripplegate 1, Canker [cancer] 1, Childbed 42, Chrisoms [a child which died in the first month of life, still wearing its baptismal chrisom-cloth] 18, Consumption 134, Convulsions 64, Cough 2, Dropsie 33, Fever 309, Flox and smallpox 5, Frighted 3, Gout 1, Grief 3, Gripes in the guts 51, Jaundices 5, Imposthume 11, Infants 16, Killed by a fall from the Bellfrey at Allhallows the Great 1, King's Evil 2, Lethargy 1, Palsie 1, Plague 7165, Rickets 17, Rising of the lights 11, Scowring [diarrhoea] 5, Scurvey 1, Spotted Fever 101, Stillborn 17, Stone and Strangury 3, Stoppage of the stomach 9, Surfeit 49, Teeth 121, Thrush 5, Tympany 1, Tissick [phthisic, a lung or throat disease] 11, Vomitting 3, Wind 3, Worms 3.

The Plague was indeed terrible, and equally lethal were many kinds of fevers, diseases such as smallpox and measles, poverty, overwork and repeated pregnancies. In Pepys' diaries he recorded that he had ten brothers and sisters, but only two survived into adulthood. According to Roy Porter in *Disease, Medicine and Society (1550-1860)*, 'the life expectancy in Stuart days was under thirty-five years'.

What were doctors able to do? Clinical examination was almost impossible due to modesty, particularly in females. Instead they had to rely on the five senses. They felt the pulse, sniffed for gangrene, tasted the urine. They could also listen for breathing irregularities, attend to the skin and eye colours and finally look for the *facies hippocratia*, the face of a dying person. As regards treatment, they advised on diet and exercise and the pursuit in all these things in moderation. In many cases there was a strong religious faith to sustain doctor and patient. There was also purging and blood letting and, of course, the use of herbs.

Georgian Times

Certainly the 18th century has been described as the Age of Enlightenment but most of the advances came from overseas and Scotland's dissenting physicians. Many of these made a great reputation in London. There was John Hunter and his brother William who worked together in the dissecting rooms. William Hunter was interested particularly in midwifery and male midwives became known as accouchers. Another well known man-midwife was William Smellie.

From across Europe came other real moves forward. Daniel Fahrenheit in 1714 produced a mercury thermometer and an Englishman, Floyer, perfected a watch for taking the pulse. In 1761 Leopold Auenbrugger, Physician-in-Chief to the Hospital of the Holy Trinity in Vienna, showed how to percuss the chest, which doctors have done ever since. Auenbrugger was, in fact, an innkeeper's son and he had been familiar since childhood with the task of striking barrels to test how full they were. Tapping with the finger ends you get different sounds from the lungs depending upon their condition, important particularly in diagnosing tuberculosis.

The microscope was developed by Leeuwenhoek of the Netherlands (1632–1723) and taken up in England by Robert Hooke. In the early days the microscope was useful particularly, for example, for looking at small insects and Dr. Muffet, whose daughter was Little Miss Muffet, made quite a name for himself with this work.

Other therapeutic advances included the detection of scurvy. The first therapeutic trial feeding fruit and vegetables was made in 1747 by Lind and proved very valuable during the voyages of Captain Cook. As usual, it was years later, in fact 1795, that the Admiralty routinely included lime and lemon juice in the Navy's diet. Other nations thought this was a bit odd, and as a result the British were called 'Limeys'. It was not known how fruit juices prevented scurvy until vitamin C was isolated in 1928.

Another advance rather nearer home came with Dr. Withering who came from Wellington in Shropshire. He was born in 1741, to a physician father, and obtained a degree in physic from the University of Edinburgh in 1766. He settled in Stafford and then Birmingham and had an interest in botanical matters, visiting Portugal. He was the first man to recognize the use of the foxglove in treating dropsy. He found that the leaves had a powerful stimulating action on the heart rhythm and increased urine flow. The therapeutic effects are due to the drug *digitalis*, although this was not isolated until much later.

Edward Jenner was an English country doctor, born in Berkeley in 1749. At the age of 13 he was sent to Mr. Daniel Ludlow of Bristol to serve an apprenticeship for six years. He married in 1788 and in 1792 obtained a degree from St. Andrews. He then became interested in the possibilities of preventing smallpox by vaccination. Jenner had learnt from the country folk in his native Gloucestershire that cowpox, a cattle disease, occasionally contracted by humans, particularly dairymaids, conferred immunity against smallpox. In 1802 Parliament granted Jenner £10,000. This summed up Jenner's success. He travelled to Vienna, Hanover, Geneva and even the United States where President Jefferson and his family were vaccinated. Napoleon also had his army vaccinated. Jenner received a degree from Oxford, and died in 1823.

The Royal Jennerian Society had been founded in 1803, but it was not until the Vaccination Act of 1853 that compulsory vaccination was introduced in Britain. Eradication by vaccination lasted in Britain right into the last century, and the World Health Organization scored a great success when, in November 1975, the last few cases in Bangladesh hit the headlines. The world's stock of vaccine has now been all but destroyed, bringing this story to a happy ending.

The first Salop Infirmary was opened in 1745 in a large house in St. Mary's Close and was extended in a very handsome new building in 1820. Meanwhile, specialist hospitals were opened in London—the maternity hospitals, and the Foundling Hospital in Bloomsbury for newborns. Mr. Coran, a retired sea captain saw, on returning from the colonies, many abandoned babies lying around the streets of London. This inspired him to build and support the Foundling Hospital.

Surgery was also rising in status and split from the Barbers in 1745. Of course, without anaesthesia operating was painful and dangerous with a high mortality risk and had to be performed with speed. William Cheselden won fame by performing a lithotomy, an operation for removal of bladder stone in two minutes flat. For this he could command huge fees, perhaps 500 guineas per patient. One of the ways in which he spent some of his money was to build a bridge over the Thames at Putney, now known as the starting point of the Boat Race.

3   John Tylston and other Whitchurch Doctors

In the 17th century, Whitchurch had three fully qualified doctors—John Tylston, Samuel Benion and Joshua Maddocks—all of whom, at some time, practised in the town. The reason why we know as much as we do about these men is due to the diaries of the remarkable dissenting clergyman, Philip Henry, and his son, Matthew.

John Tylston's father lived in Alkington, near Whitchurch and died in 1684. John Tylston himself was probably born in Whitchurch on 15th March 1661. After leaving school he resided with the Reverend Mr. Malden in Alkington, and perfected his skill in Greek and Hebrew. After Malden's death he was admitted to Trinity College, Oxford and took a degree in Natural Philosophy. He then moved to London where he studied under Sir Richard Blackmore and his fame reached the learned Dr. Sydenham, who, according to Matthew Henry's diary, admitted him to his circle of friends.

In 1687 Tylston obtained a degree in Physic from the University of Aberdeen which, incidentally, was the first university in northern Europe to establish a medical school. Dr. Tylston then established his professional career in Whitchurch and married Katherine, the second daughter of the Reverend Philip Henry, at Whitewell Chapel, near Whitchurch.

In 1690 Tylston moved to practise in Chester. In 1696 the Reverend Philip Henry became ill and according to Matthew Henry 'Dr. Tylston and I attended him possibly with a kidney stone'. Philip Henry died on 24th June, Midsummer-day, in the same year, at the age of 65 and was buried in St. Alkmund's Church. John Tylston wrote his epitaph which is contained on a plaque in the church. John Tylston himself died on 8th April 1699 in his 35th year. His son, Thomas Tylston, became a Doctor of Physic, as did his grandson, John, who became a Physician at Chester Infirmary in 1755.

Some of John Tylston's views have come down to us in a book called *The Country Physician*, a copy of which is preserved in the British Library. Catalogued under John Tylston's name, it was issued by an anonymous

THE

COUNTRY

PHYSICIAN;

Containing feveral eafie and ufeful Remedies, fome whereof were never
made publick before, with fome fhort
Advices tending to Health.

AS ALSO

Several Letters lately writen by an E-
minent Phyfician, to the Publifher.

By a well-wifher to the Art of Phyfick, and the
Health of his Country-men.

EDINBURGH,
Printed in the Year, M. DCC. L

PREFACE

TO THE

READER.

HEALTH *is a great Bleffing; and a
found Mind in a found Body is a
great Happinefs: for when mens
flefh upon them is in pain, it makes their
Souls within them to mourn. Health is
of the moft comfortable importance, next
unto the Salvation of the Souls of men,
efpecially when we confider what a mul-
titude of Diftempers the mortal Bodies of
men are expofed unto. If men did but
confider the wonderfull Compofure of
their Bodies, the Situation of their Parts,
the Circulation of the Bloud, the feveral Meanders of the Veins, Arteries and
Nerves,*

Two of the opening pages to The Country Physician

publisher in Edinburgh in 1750. It includes three letters written and signed
by Tylston between 1695 and 1698, the book's introduction reading:

> Containing several easy and useful remedies, some whereof were
> never made public before, with some short advices tending to health.
> Also several letters lately written by an eminent physician to the
> publisher.

The book then moves on to 56 Herbal Remedies, of which the following are
a selection:

For the Jaundice
Take a handful of Chickenweed, cut it small, and infuse the same in
a mutchkin of white Wine. Let the infusion stand twenty four hours,
then pour off the clear liquor, and drink the one half thereof in the
morning, and the other half at four in the afternoon: repeat this for
three days together.

For Bleeding at the Nose

Take half a mutchkin of Vinegar, and dissolve therein an ounce of Sugar of Lead (called in Latin *Saccharum Saturni*) and then take a Linen cloth doubled, and dip it in the cold liquor, and apply it to the Breast, and renew the application as often as the cloth begins to warm.

If all else fails for bleeding of the nose -
Take a Plaister of Potters Clay, mix with Vinegar, and the white of an Egg, and apply it to the Testicles. Or let the Patient that Bleedeth, chew the root of a Nettle in his mouth, but not swallow it down.

For a Woman in Labour

Take the Livers of Eels and reduce to Powder, a drop weight: give it in a glass of White or Menish Wine well sweetened with Sugar: there is nothing better to facilitate Delivery.

For the Toothache

Take a good quantity of Tobacco, and boil it in a mutchkin of white Wine very strong; take a little of it hot, and hold it in your mouth till the strength of it be gon, and spit out the Phlegm, do so till the pain be passed, but warm the Wine when you take it: Take heed none goes over your Throat, for it will make you Sick.

In the first letter written by John Tylston he writes:

> ... I was lately called to a woman in White-church, who had for many years laboured under a violent Flux Menftr. with excessive pains: she had the advice of severals and particularly of a very ingenious physician of my acquaintance. The mean methods of absorbent and astringent remedies, milk, diet &c. had been sufficiently tried without effect. I prescribed a Merc. compound, to be taken every morning in an Emulsion, sweetened with Diacodium, for about a week together, which put her into a salvation, almost as plentiful, and lasting, as what we commonly obtain by Unguent, took off her pains and Flux, and perfectly cured her, without any other administration.
>
> The success of Dr.Sydenham's method in Fevers is a subject too large to be touched upon now in the end of a letter ...

This first letter was written in Chester, on 16th October 1695. In the second letter, written in Chester on Christmas Eve that same year, he discusses:

... In diseases that are of an inflamatory nature, in which it is generally as hard to remove them, as it is easy to prevent them, if due care be taken in time I have used pigeons with admirable success in other fevers, applying them dissected to the feet in Phrenfy, alive to the anus in convulsions &c. But this fever laughs at such applications ...

In Dr. Tylston's final letter written in Chester, dated 18th February 1698, he writes of:

The indiscrete and promiscuous use of the bath-waters (now too much in vogue) hath been fatal to many. The drinking of them is very useful to some that are of cold phlegmatic constitution, whose blood is much enriched thereby, but as for those that have a hot fermenting blood, that is of a plethorick nature, it makes it very mischievous to them.

A famous instance (after many others) I met with this winter, in a person of great worth and figure in Lancashire, that hath been my patient for some years. He is of a thin habit of body and hath sharp colerick blood.

This gentleman was last summer earnestly persuaded to the bath by some at London. I positively forbad it, for the reasons above-mentioned, however he went and drank the water, but from that time his blood took a fret, and grew very unquiet. I cured him at the expense of letting off about forty ounces of blood and frequent purges and he became very weak and wasted. However, in a fortnight's time, to my admiration, he recovered from extreme weakness and went out hunting.

At the end of the letters he states 'The Powder of Afarum, used as you advised, hath been of very great use to many here, against deafness or difficulty of hearing, particularly to the Bishop of Chester. I have prescribed it to others with good success, and I doubt not it may be equally beneficial in many other Cephalick affections.'

The other two afore-mentioned doctors in Whitchurch who were contemporaries of Tylston were Joshua Maddocks and Samuel Benion. Maddocks obtained a BA degree from Cambridge in 1660. According to the St. Alkmund's *Parish Magazine* the Revd. George Eyre Evans reported in 1893 as follows:

There was Dr. Joshua Maddocks 'a beloved physician' and 'very dear friend and kindsman' of Philip Henry, who lamented the death of his friend, of a fever, at Whitchurch on 27th July 1682.

To quote Matthew Henry:

> Dr. Samuel Benion was born in Whixall, in the parish of Prees, on 14th June 1673 His mother was the daughter of Richard Sadler, a worthy nonconformist minister, who was turned out from Ludlow by the Act of Uniformity. The Rev. Mr. Sadler died in 1675, and Samuel Benion was baptized by his grandfather.
>
> He began his learning with the schoolmaster at Whixall but in 1688 was removed to the free-school at Wirksworth in Derbyshire where he remained until he was eighteen.
>
> In 1691 he went to live with Philip Henry at Broad Oak, near Whixall, who employed him in teaching other gentlemen's sons. In 1692 he moved to London where he had the opportunity of hearing the best preachers. In June 1695 he began studying at Glasgow University and in May 1696 took a degree of Master of Arts. Returning to his family house in Whixall at the age of twenty-three he began to preach first at Broad Oak and then at the small chapel in Dodington. He also set up at Higher Farm an 'Academy of Learning' where he took on the tutorage of as many as thirty nonconformists.
>
> In 1703, at the suggestion of his mother, he went back to Glasgow and took a degree in Physic. In November that year he married Grace Yates, a daughter of Thomas Yates of Dearnford, near Whitchurch, by whom he had two sons. He was particularly interested in mathematics and natural philosophy and although he lived in obscurity he found the means to acquaint himself with modern discoveries.

In his final years Dr. Benion went to live in Shrewsbury. On Monday 23rd February 1708, he complained a little of pain in his back and head. He died on 4th March, aged 34, and was buried in St. Chad's Church in Shrewsbury.

Local doctors in Georgian times

The very first Medical Register of 1783 contains the names of doctors all over Britain. The list is divided into doctors who attended a university and obtained a degree in physic, and doctors who obtained a licence from a bishop to practice as surgeon/apothecaries. Other doctors also appear on the list in this register but there is no note as to their qualifications.

Concerning Whitchurch, the list contains details of Dr. Bennion who received a degree in physic from Glasgow University in 1703, and Edward Wicksteed who received a licence in the same year from the Bishop of Lambeth. The other doctors in Whitchurch had, as far as we know, been trained on an apprentice basis as surgeon/apothecaries. There was the partnership of Wicksteed and Meakin, and the individuals John Brookes and Edward Jones.

In her 'great journeys' of 1698 around England and Wales Celia Fiennes noted in her diary on her visit to Whitchurch: 'This is a large market town, here are two very fine gardens, one belongs to an apothecary [thought to have been Edward Wicksteed] full of all fruits and greens. The other was at the Crown Inn where I staid'. Edward Wicksteed died in 1711.

Richard Wicksteed was almost certainly Edward's son and he became a 'master', meaning that he had apprentices. At one stage he had eight of them, each having to pay £80 a year for seven years' training, so it was big business. He was also known to own Ye Olde Crowne Inn in 1761, and was listed as a subscriber to Simon Mason's *Practical Observations in Physick*.

Francis Bostock lived at Bostock Hall in Whixall and became a surgeon/apothecary in 1708. He consulted at The Red Lyon, Whitchurch High Street. In 1715 he became a master, charging £10 a year for seven years' training and he had three apprentices: John Rutland, John Jole and Robert Sidwell. There is an interesting tale about 'Dr. Bostock, Dr. of Physic' who must have had a high reputation from the entries in a diary of the early 18th century. The story begins at Ince-Blundell Hall, outside Liverpool, where Sir Nicholas Blundell had a wife who needed attention for a bad back, and failing to get satisfaction from local doctors, they decided to travel to Whitchurch to consult Dr. Bostock.

> Aug. 18th 1709 - my wife and I began our journey towards Whitchurch but came too late for ye bote at Liverpool, so went over at Runk Horn (Runcorn), after which we lost our way and got a guide that brought us to Frodsham, at the 'Sign of Ye Bear's Paw'.
> Aug-19th - we went from there to Whitchurch at the 'Sign of Ye Red Lyon' - where we dined and discussed with Dr. Bostock about my wife's paine in her back. ...

Sir Nicholas also wanted physic for the children which cost 15s., so that it was an expensive trip, with the doctor's fee of £1 1s. 6d., plus travelling charges of £1 4s. 11d. It is not recorded whether his 'wife's paines' were alleviated, but in any case a trip of 40 miles each way on rough roads would not help.

A local historian, R.B. James, lists many other surgeon/apothecaries over the course of the 18th century. John Nettles worked around 1689; Tristan Daxon was a master in 1713; William Roe became an apprentice in 1729 and then subsequently a master in 1748; William Woodrich worked between 1740 and 1764; Richard Redrope was a master who died in 1743 (who charged £22 a year for seven years' training); and Paul Figes was the son of Robert Roe, a butcher in Whitchurch.

The other noted surgeon/apothecary was Thomas Higgins of Wem. He was described as an early provincial 'man-midwife'. In London William Smellie published *The Theory and Practice of Midwifery* sometime between 1752 and 1764. Men who were qualified as surgeons increasingly took on some midwifery work, and by the end of the 18th century men were retained as midwives throughout the provinces. What started out as the fashionable option for wealthy women quickly became the routine even for ordinary people. Certainly, by the end of the century it was common for surgeon/apothecaries to undertake some obstetrical work.

Over the years 1781 to 1803 Thomas Higgins kept a register containing information of 1,200 births which he and his father had attended. He gave the parents' names, addresses, dates of birth and whether they were born alive or dead. These records were made in order to bill patients for his services and did not contain any clinical information, except for noting an occasional twin pregnancy and a single use of forceps when, on 21st August 1788, he delivered a girl, born alive. It may be, of course, that he used forceps on other occasions without making a specific entry in the register.

On 3rd May 1796 he attended three separate births, one at 11 am, one at 12 noon, and one between 2 pm and 3 pm. He and his father also continued the usual work of surgeon/apothecaries doing minor surgery such as setting bones, pulling teeth, bleeding and inoculation against smallpox (for the latter charging 5 shillings for adults and half a crown for each child). They also dispensed a detailed list of drugs including ointments, drops, purges and liniment.

His standard or lowest fee for attendance at births was 10s. 6d. but he took into account the means of the parents and, in some cases, charged up to 2 guineas or even 3 guineas. He also treated some clients whom he described as paupers, some of them under the care of the overseers of the poor in Wem, who were charged the lowest rate.

Thomas Higgins died prematurely at the age of 44. After his death in 1803 his probate inventory shows that he was a keen sportsman, possessing pistols and other guns, fishing rods and even a sword. His good quality furniture included a mahogany tea-urn stand. He lived the life of a middle-class household making a prosperous career out of his skill and earnings.

4   Deermoss Hospital – The House of Industry

After Henry VIII closed the monasteries there were two ways in which the sick and destitute could be helped. One was by private charity, the other was by a state-organized system which was the first in Europe.

Those who adhered to Christian principles, or who were socially minded, began to give money to help the poor either by occasional hand-outs on special occasions, or more particularly on their deathbeds and through wills. Many charities were endowed, for instance, there was the Higginson Trust in Whitchurch, and the big country estates also gave generously to the poor. In addition, Trade Guilds were formed, one of their roles being to look after their members in their old age.

After 1689 the Established Church and dissenting groups had their own charities. The running of these establishments were put together in terms which were designed to foster piety and the observance of Christian worship. Good behaviour was an essential condition and the concept of helping the deserving poor, but not the undeserving, was very much in mind.

In the 17th century new hospitals sprung up, first in London and other big cities and by 1800 all sizable towns had their own hospital. The first Salop Infirmary was opened in 1745 in a large house in St. Mary's Close and was extended in a very handsome new building in 1820. These hospitals were worked on what was called the 'voluntary system', where people who could afford it paid and poorer people were treated free with money raised through charities.

The state was also at work. In 1597, during the reign of Elizabeth I, the government placed the responsibility of caring for the poor on each parish. There followed many Acts of Parliament which defined the wishes of central government but this was not always locally enforced. The people in charge at the lowest level were parish officers: churchwardens, overseers of the poor and constables. At a district level Justices of the Peace enforced the policies and at Quarter Sessions they received the Privy Council orders. The operation of the Poor Law was fundamental to every community, from at least the mid 16th century. Local government took care of the sick and orphans and attended to matters of public health.

In Whitchurch, for example, in April 1636 the Manor Court confirmed a series of laws concerned with public health, the sale of food and drink, and fire precautions in a document called a *Payne Book*. This lists 68 laws to be obeyed 'on payne' to pay penalties ranging from one shilling to 40 shillings.

For instance: No-one was to put any dung, entrails or any other ordure into any ditch, pool or pit to the annoyance of the inhabitants—on 'payne' of 6s. 8d. No hemp or flax should be washed in any running stream, for which there was a penalty for non compliance of 20s. All water courses and ditches were to be kept clean, on a similar penalty of 20s. The street in front of the market had to be swept at least once a week and the muck and soil disposed of—on 'payne' of 1s. Innkeepers must not sell less than one full quart of best beer or ale for 1d., or suffer a penalty of 13s. 4d. Householders had to supply fire-fighting equipment such as buckets, ladders, long hooks and brazen squirts—a kind of stirrup pump. The town constable inspected the equipment once a quarter, the penalty for any neglect being 10s.

By 1611 each parish had to provide a 'house of habitation' for its own poor. In Whitchurch a property in Newtown had been used as a Poor House but after many years use it was in a bad condition.

In 1790 an Act was made to allow inspection of Poor or Work Houses, on a warrant from Justices of the Peace, by surgeons, physicians, apothecaries and officiating clergy. This allowed the examination of premises to help prevent the spread of contagious diseases, or where the inadequate provision of clothing, bedding etc. were suspected, or where a complaint had been made.

It wasn't long before the Act was applied to inspect the Whitchurch premises, and in January 1791 Mr. J. Scottock, Clerk of Works, gave the following reasons for condemning the old Poor Law premises:

> The buildings for the reception of the poor of the parish of Whitchurch in the County of Salop are situated in the town of Whitchurch and consist of two small houses (A and C), a room called the lower house (K) and a building originally erected for the water works marked (B).
>
> There are at present 60 men, women and children in these buildings, and I am informed by the person who farms the poor that he pays 140 paupers besides.
>
> The room marked (K) is timber, thatched and very very old as well as out of repair, adjoining is the privy and pigsty which is offensive. The garden contains one fourth of an acre.

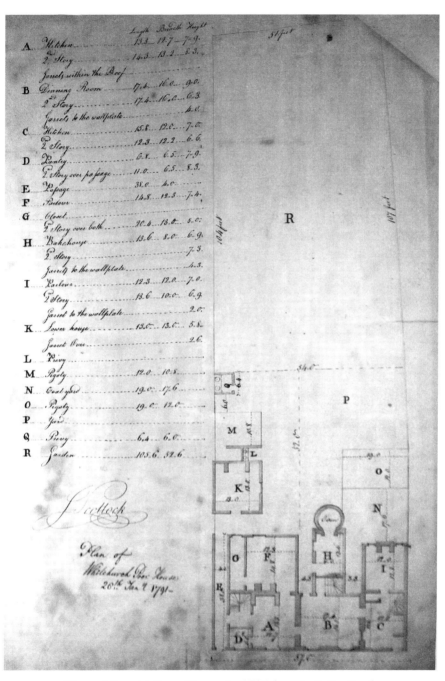

*Plan of the old Poor House in 1791 by Mr. J. Scottock,
which he then condemned*

29

For these reasons I am of the opinion that the said buildings will not admit of such alterations and additions as will obviate the inconveniences complained of.

In April 1791 there followed a further report:

> I examined some of the men. They were dirty and their clothes lousy. The linen on their beds was offensive. The rooms were not kept clean and being too small emitted a very noisome effluvia.
>
> No attention is paid to the ventilation of the House. The apartments called the Lower House have not been repaired and rains in on a pauper when in bed.
>
> The filth of the chamber pots are thrown promiscuously about.
>
> The yard and the whole house is badly conducted. The Rev. N. Collier, Mr. Moakin, surgeon and Mr. Jones, surgeon attended the Poor House and can give further information relating to this business.

There was concern to replace the existing establishment, and during 1791 the Reverend Francis Henry Egerton took a lively interest in steering a local Act of Parliament required to set up a new House of Industry. In the Rector's book St. Alkmund's Church there are letters written in his own handwriting, with his views on how the Act could work.

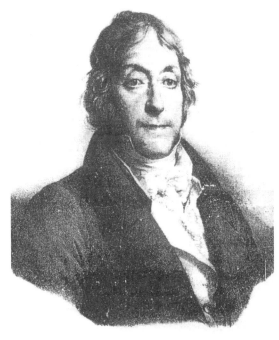

Francis Henry Egerton

Egerton was one of life's eccentrics. Born in 1756 he had a brilliant academic career, becoming a Bachelor of Arts aged 20, a Master of Arts and Fellow of All Souls at 24, and a Fellow of the Royal Society at 25. He was ordained when 24 and became Rector of Whitchurch and Myddle when 25 in 1781. He enjoyed the life of a county squire, hunting and shooting on the estates. Yet he dressed his dogs up like human beings and many of them had a place at his table so long as they did not misbehave. He was keen on litigation. His most famous lawsuit was against the barrister, Wickstead, whom he had tormented with a bizarre system of a tethered fox barking like a dog, fixed to a bell, and a wind driven propeller attached to a rattle which made a continuous noise in a field next to Wickstead's house. This cost him much in damages. He spent the last 26 years of his life as an absentee parson, living in London and Paris, and employed three curates to look after his churches. He never married and although a cleric had five illegitimate children, all girls. The last child, Sarah Cotton, lived with him for most of his life. During his last few years he became the eighth Earl of Bridgewater; the Duke of Bridgewater (the Canal Duke) was his cousin. With this position he came into even more money, and on his death in 1803 he donated some of the contents of the Bridgewater library at Ashridge to the British Museum, which have become known as the Egerton Collection. He also donated £2,000 for the relief of the poor in Whitchurch and Myddle.

The Act of Parliament was passed and in 1794 Deermoss Hospital was built as a House of Industry on a greenfield site, on a hill, outside the town. Its architect, Mr. W. Turner was another interesting character. He was working under Telford on the building of the Ellesmere and Llangollen canals at about the same time as he put forward the plans for the House of Industry. Turner had also re-designed the Rector's house and his plans included a water closet which would probably have been the first in the town. His plans for Deermoss Hospital were as follows:

House of Industry to consist of:

> principal floor 11 ft high
> bed chamber floor 10 ft high
> attic 9 ft high

Ground Floor and Cellar:

> Boardroom for the court of Directors
> Kitchen
> parlour
> storeroom
> pantry and larder
> scullery
> washroom and bakehouse
> laundry
> two small rooms for temporary confinements
> diningroom to accommodate 100 poor

workroom for men and boys
workroom for women and girls
schoolroom of sufficient dimensions to receive the whole
family for the morning and evening prayer

Bed chamber floor

twenty separate lodging rooms to hold one bed each
four wards for men, women, boys and girls that will
conveniently hold 10 beds each. The beds to be no nearer
than 4ft to each other, nor nearer than 8ft to each other end
to end
two storerooms
three bed chambers for governors, matron and servant

Offices and the Sick Quarters - detached:

Two wards for sick - 5 beds each for males and females
Bed chambers for Attendants
Bath with both warm and cold water
Room to receive dead bodies
This building is to be not nearer than 60ft to the house.

Other buildings on site:

Coal house
midding with proper drains
pigsty
courtyard

A separate chapel was not built until 1882 when it was opened by the Bishop of Lichfield.

The original stone inscription was incorporated into the wall of the building and its contents stated 'This House intended for the relief and comfort of the poor of this parish was built in the year of our Lord MDCCXC1V'. This stone is now positioned in the wall near the front entrance of the new hospital.

The House of Industry was managed by 12 directors or guardians who nominated a chairman. These constituted a board of regulation of the work-house and the paupers belonging to the 14 townships of Whitchurch. The guardians met weekly to review progress and give out punishment.

When completed the building could accommodate 150 inmates, but on its opening the number on the books was 63. The staff consisted of a master,

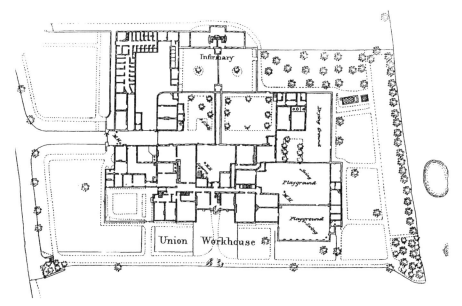

Plan of the Workhouse in 1880

often a joint appointment with his wife, and there were other servants including nurses and even a schoolmistress.

The children knitted socks, the women washed, spun and wove, the men gardened, cobbled and farmed. They received no wages, only gratuities, and each 'stopt' for any breach of the rules was recorded. If a man or woman was hired out their wages were paid to the overseer. Occasionally, they were allowed to retain some of their 'earnings', for example Elizabeth Shakeshaft 'spinning one lb of linen yarn out of house' was given 4½d, and three children 5d. in total for knitting socks.

Flax was generally bought in 30lbs lots at a time, and after spinning was sold to local tradesmen. Sometimes House of Industry products were sold openly in the market: '15th May 1796 paid Mr. Richard Corser, Treasurer, for 204 ells of cloth sold at Whitchurch fair £10. 1s. 11d.'.

Shoemaking took up a lot of the inmates' time. In the account books there is an entry 'made 22 pairs of shoes for £1. 2s. 5d.' It is not clear if this was the total sum for the shoes.

Ann Dulson received a gratuity of 4d. for making handkerchiefs, seven aprons and associated mending. Clearly the aim of the House of Industry was to be as self supporting as possible.

Apart from the payments to butchers, the occasional goose and milk, the only other outside payments were for raw materials.

The account book is also revealing in other ways. For the ten year period following its opening (1795–1805) it provides some interesting information abut the lives of the inmates. It showed that it provided a refuge for illegitimate children—the charge was 1s. 6d. per half year, and that the children were baptized not by a clergyman but by the church clerk, at 6d. a head. Periodically the record mentions a guinea paid to the parson for 'searching the Church registers for the ages of 20 children'. The house also acted as a form of labour exchange as denoted by the entry of a payment in 1796 'to Eliz Namer to carry her and her daughter to Bangor where she hired her daughter to Mr. Parsons for 30s. per annum'.

Occasionally some single service by an inmate would be rewarded by the Court of Directors: 'Thos. Jenkin for his care and attention of the cow and calves 1s.'. For the rest it was left to the overseer to punish or reward as he saw fit. He paid the schoolmistress 3d. weekly. Richard Taylor earned 6d. for sitting up all night with Sarah Savage. 'To Eliz Lea and Matty Horton 1d. for tobacco for laying out the corpse of Eliz Sandford'. 'To four men and a cart from Alkington Hall for bringing a lunatic to the House of Industry 5s.'. 'To flannel for Marg Adams to make a shift for Salvation, ordered by Mr. James 3s. 1½d.'.

Examples of recorded Punishments in 1805 are as follows: 'Tea and Sugar to Mary Welsh stopt nine times for misbehaviour in throwing her victuals on the hall floor'. 'To Thos. Williams for coming to put Will Horton, Martha Horton and J. Bellingham in ye crib for fighting - 6d.'. 'Gratuity to Sam Kempster stopt this week on account of his having gone to town without leave for a day and a night and coming home drunk and very abusive'.

The more serious crimes were reported to the Court of Directors and some went to Shrewsbury.

In the years following the opening of the hospital, Mr. Edward Jones, surgeon and physician, was available for consultation and prescriptions. One such prescription for a fever, regardless of the patient's age or sex, was a wig. On 17th January 1797 there is the record 'to a wig for Thos Darlington ill in ye fever, ½d'—he died a week later aged 4 years old.

Elsewhere in the account book is noted: 'to a quart of vinegar for Ann Meashon's room, tar and gunpowder ordered by Mr. Jones to correct the air - 10d'. However poor Ann died soon afterwards in spite of the fumigation.

Tea was the general panacea for ills, but occasionally sugar: 'to ½lb of sugar for growel for the sick people - 1s. 3d.'.

One Richard Sutton who came into the house by order of Mr. Hassall, arrived with 'the itch'—result ½lb hog's lard to mix with sulphur sent by Mr. Jones to rub on it. Eliz Phithias' 'gammy' knee was treated as follows:

Quarter pint of brandy 7d. to be mixed with 2oz of best Florentine oil 5d. and white bread for poultices'.

The more serious cases were sent to the Royal Salop Infirmary. Margaret Adams' journey there was recorded for 10th February 1797: 'Paid Matron's waggoner for taking Margaret Adams to Salop Infirmary where she went on Tuesday morning in care of Matron Fox - 2s. To expenses on road for breakfast. and dinner - 1s. 5d., for 4 night lodging for the said M. Adams, ordered by the surgeon, there being no bed for her until Saturday morning - 6s.'.

The accounts showed at frequent intervals in the overseer's scholarly hand: 'to Beer for ourselves - 3s. 6d.'.

Prees also had its own Poor House and there are some interesting records regarding two medical men in 1729, Mr. Roe and Mr. Holbrook, presumably surgeon/apothecaries. Holbrook was awarded 9 shillings from parish funds for being 'in want', and his daughter Sarah received a pauper's funeral in the same year. About that time Roe also appeared to be in receipt of Poor Law help. It would seem that doctors did not have a method of regular payment from the overseers, or if so, the amount needed was not enough.

However, in 1774 the Prees Vestry came to an agreement with two Whitchurch doctors, Mr. Tomkinson, surgeon, and Mr. Meakin, apothecary, to supply paupers belonging to Prees who would be sent by the churchwardens or overseers for physic or surgery, (midwifery excepted). Some of their itemised bills survive in the Vestry Minutes Book. The following series of entries for 1775 show some of the help given:

April 21st	John Gaugh's wife when lying in	£00 : 02 : 00
24th	John Gaugh's being ill	£00 : 04 : 00
27th	for a shoulder of veal for John Gaugh's wife, she being ill	£00 : 01 : 06
29th	coals for John Gaugh	£00 : 01 : 06
	neck of mutton for John Gaugh's wife	£00 : 01 : 00
May 3rd	John Gaugh's wife, she being ill	£00 : 02 : 00
5th	John Gaugh's wife, she being ill	£00 : 01 : 00
10th	neck of mutton for Gaugh's wife	£00 : 01 : 00
	Andrew Jackson for making Gaugh's children clothes	£00 : 02 : 00
	Little gown for Gaugh's child	£00 : 01 : 00
23rd	Mary Collins for laying Gaugh's wife	£00 : 05 : 00

The story does not end happily. Later in the month there are charges for laying out Gaugh's wife, for a coffin and for the burial fees. In March the following year there is a charge for a coffin for Gaugh's child.

The following is an itemised bill for treatment supplied:

July 19th 1780

	Delivering Mary Ratcliff	£1 : 01 : 00
	Attendance upon Gough's wife in labour	£1 : 01 : 00
	Innoculating 11 poor children at the workhouse	£1 : 07 : 06
	Year's attendance upon the poor of Prees	£9 : 09 : 00
	Total	£12 : 18 : 06

There are numerous entries in every year for financial help given to people 'in sickness'. There are other entries of a more specific nature.

1775
May 25th   Peter Taylor to have his teeth drawn   £00 : 00 : 02

What story lies behind this entry?

1794
March   Doctor's bill for fracture upon the head
of George Blanthorn   £9 : 09 : 00

There are several instances of food and drink being given in sickness.

1773   Prees Quarter
For a bottle of Daffey's for widow
in her illness   £00 : 01 : 03
1775   Whixall Quarter
paid for wine for Widow Chidlow   £00 : 01 : 00
1795   Sandford Quarter paid for wine for
Sergeant's wife by order of Dr. Jones   £00 : 05 : 01

In the first *Whitchurch Herald* in 1869 the following notice was published:

WHITCHURCH UNION

The Guardians of the Poor of the Whitchurch Union will, at their MEETING to be held on Friday, the 16th April next, proceed to the Appointment of NURSE to the Workhouse, at a Salary of £16 per annum, with full Rations, Washing and Lodgings.

The Nurse appointed must be between the ages of 25 and 50, without incumbrance, and must be prepared, when unoccupied with her duties to the sick, to make herself generally useful in assisting the Matron.

Applications, with Testimonials of character and fitness, to be sent on or before the 15th April, to me,

R.B. Jones

Clerk to the Guardians

There are also on record contracts for provisions at the Whitchurch Union dated 8th March 1869, and for a schoolmistress at a salary of £20 per annum dated 12th February 1869.

There were known to be 103 inmates of the Workhouse in 1877, a year in which Christmas was celebrated in the following manner. At 9 a.m. Divine Service was held in the dining room, led by the chaplain, the Revd. J.C. Harris. At 12.30 p.m. dinner was served, the menu consisting of beef followed by plum pudding. At 6 p.m. tea and plumcake was served, and at 7 p.m. the inmates met in the dining room and spent a couple of hours in 'harmless mirth'. They were given their usual allowance of ale and the toast was proposed by a member of the Board of Guardians. There then followed songs, together with music provided by the band of the Whitchurch Rifle Volunteers.

The following was composed and sung by a visitor to Whitchurch about 1880:

We've all had a rattling feast to-day
Well worthy of Christmas time,
And each of us thought, if he did not say
By Jingo! but isn't it prime!
It could be no other for Bradbury's beef
Is noted the country round.
And the happiest man in this room to-night
Is the man who has eaten two pound.

From the uproar you're making I think it is clear
The dinners made some of you ill;
And if in the morning you still feel queer
Go and ask Dr. George for a pill.
He keeps a good store in his surgery drawer
And take them as free as you will,
Christmas gifts are in season and for that same reason
He won't put them down in his bill.

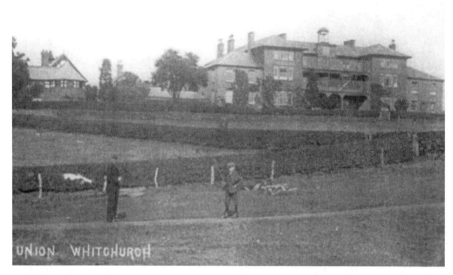

Deermoss Hospital in about 1920

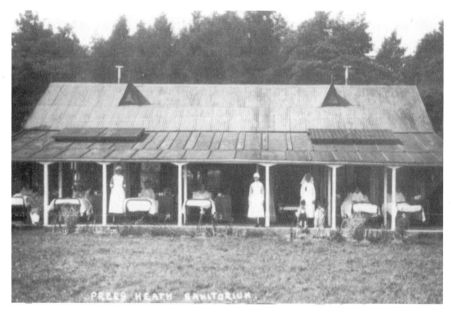

Prees Heath Isolation Hospital

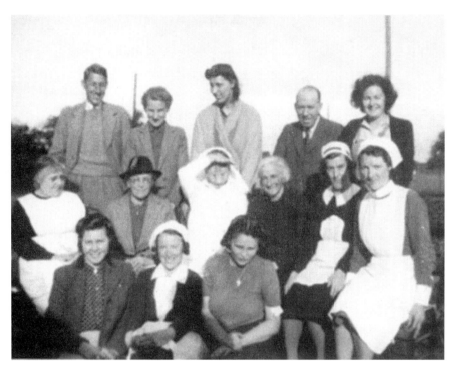

A photograph of the staff of the Isolation Hospital,
including the doctors and the matron

In 1909 a Royal Commission reported on its inquiry into the Poor Law. The Commission felt that the Boards of Guardians had outlived their usefulness and could be swept away, and that the terms 'workhouse' and 'pauper' should no longer be used. Administration was passed to local government, and in 1930 the county council took over the running of the hospital until 1949, when it became part of the National Health Service.

As regards other community facilities there was an Isolation Hospital opened on Prees Heath in 1903, used mainly for tuberculosis patients. The doctors in attendance there were Dr. Elliott, Dr. Brown, Dr. Mitchell and Dr. Franklin.

Mrs. Perry has given me information and photographs of the Isolation Hospital where she was a patient for a year in 1944. She remembers she was there for her 21st birthday and the staff made her a cake. She says there were two wards of four beds each and a verandah of ten beds. The mainstay of treatment was fresh air and some drugs. Dr. Somerset of Wem was looking after her. She remembers another patient who was a landgirl.

The Isolation Hosptal made a great contribution to medical care during the time of its operation when tunerculosis and other infectious diseases were rife.

The hospital is now converted into kennels.

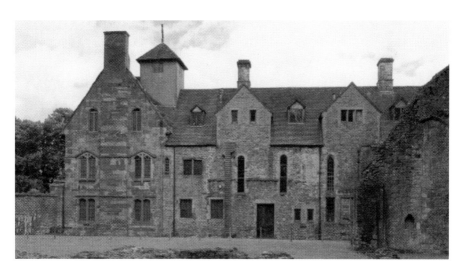

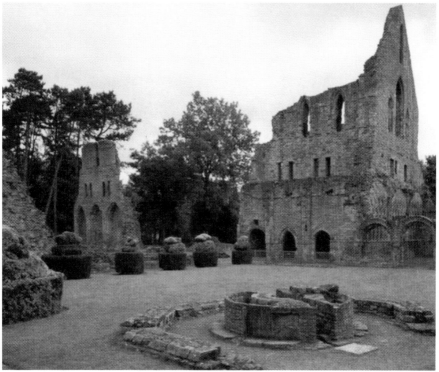

Wenlock Priory Infirmary (above) and Lavatorium (below, foreground)

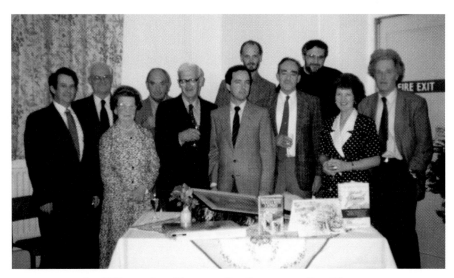

Dr. Wilson, Dr. Clayton, Dr. Rogerson, Dr. Flewett,
Dr. Thompson, Dr. Terry, Dr. Giles, Dr. Teather, Mr. Blunt,
Matron Blackmore and Sister Miller

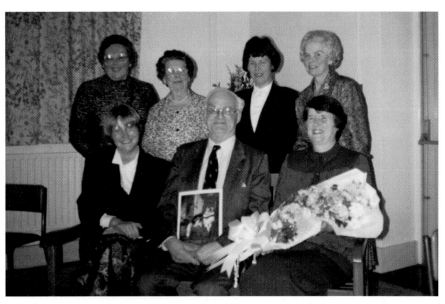

Photograph taken on my retirement in 1987. Back row, from left to right:
Sister Barbara Williams, Matron Blackmore, Kay Casbolt
and Mrs. Hutton. Front row: My daughter Dr. Ruth Clayton, myself
and my wife, Judith

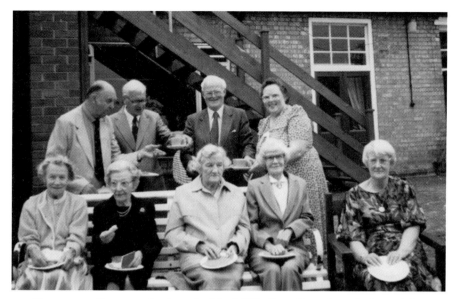

*Centenary Party at the hospital in 1997. Standing, from left to right:
Dr. Rogerson, Dr. Flewett, myself and Sister Barbara Williams. Seated:
Mrs. Hatton, Nurse Cadman, Mrs. Lee, Mrs. Worrall and Nurse Johnson*

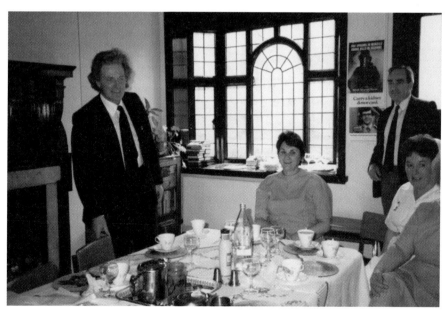

*A small party after the last operating session at the hospital showing
Mr. Blunt, Dr. Giles and nursing staff*

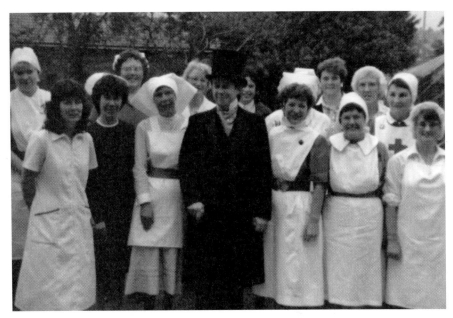

Anniversary of the building of the hospital in 1886, with Dr. Paul Wilson and members of staff in uniforms of years gone by

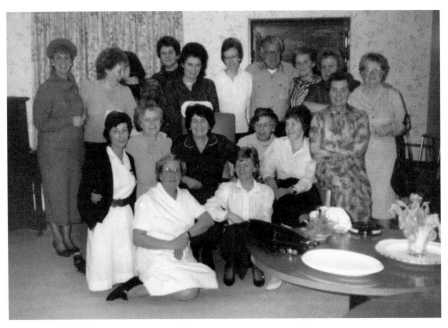

A picture of Deermoss staff

5   Victorian England

Even the earliest societies, certainly from 2000 BC, were aware of the deadening qualities of opium, hashish and alcohol and these were fully used whenever surgical procedures were possible. However, it was in the Victorian era that real advances in surgical care were made. The reason for this was anaesthesia, an expression coined by an American, Oliver Wendell Holmes, to indicate the effects of ether.

The next 'sleeping' gas discovered was nitrous oxide, which Humphrey Davy found induced dizziness and relaxation of muscles and a tendency to laugh, hence its popular name. Both ether and nitrous oxide were used in America as an anaesthetic for dental extractions.

In January 1847 James Young Simpson of Edinburgh first used chloroform to relieve the pains of childbirth and it began to be used extensively for this purpose. Queen Victoria received chloroform, administered by John Snow, for the birth of Prince Leopold in 1853. The Queen was delighted, feeling it 'soothing, quietening and delightful beyond measure' as she wrote in her Journal.

The other big risk after surgery was post-operative infection. Joseph Lister was a Quaker and became Professor of Surgery at Glasgow Royal Infirmary in 1861. He knew about Louis Pasteur's work on bacteria and concluded that the best way to control wound infection and putrefaction was to use carbolic soap lint in the dressings, and later he advocated carbolic sprays.

As early as 1874 Louis Pasteur had suggested passing instruments through boiling water or through a flame, and heat sterilization was quickly accepted for instruments. In 1890, at the John Hopkins University in America, rubber gloves, face masks and surgical gowns were used for the first time. As a result of these developments in hygiene operations were more successful. In 1901, just before his Coronation, Edward VII was operated on for an appendicectomy.

Many country practitioners had acquired medical degrees from Edinburgh and Glasgow and a few from the newly founded London University, and the 1858 Medical Act led to the formation of the General Medical Council. The British Medical Association (BMA) grew up as a ginger group of doctors from the provinces.

In spite of all these varied advances the average GP in England found that the going was pretty tough. They were very over-worked and on call all hours, and had to be endlessly civil to the snobby, affluent patients, whilst coping with slow payers and bad debts. Many took jobs as Poor Law doctors in workhouses, earning possibly £200 a year. However, in some county towns like Winchester, practitioners did quite well attending as physicians to local voluntary hospitals. The Whitchurch doctors I have researched seemed to have been comfortable with their households and their high standing in their own community.

Another great improvement in patient care was that nursing became professional, largely due to the efforts of Florence Nightingale and Elizabeth Fry. They both trained at the Deaconess Institute established near Düsseldorf in Germany. On Elizabeth Fry's return to England she founded the Institute of Nursing. Florence Nightingale, coming from a comfortable, wealthy background, discovered nursing as an outlet for her energies and desire to help the sick poor. In the Crimean War of 1854-56 the sick and wounded were looked after by untrained male orderlies, but Florence Nightingale arrived at the Barrack Hospital of Scutari on the Black Sea and within six months, in the face of considerable opposition, had transformed the place. With the right background and contacts in London to get the equipment that she needed, the death rate fell from 40% to 2%. On her return to England she organized the new St. Thomas's Hospital in London, opposite the Houses of Parliament, and started the Nightingale Schools which spread all over the British Empire.

Another improvement was made by a Swedish Banker, Jean Henri Dunant, who saw the horrors of war between French and Italian forces and he started the International Red Cross in 1864.

Local Doctors
Amongst the local doctors Dr. John Brookes was classified as a surgeon/apothecary in the first Medical Register of 1783. He was known to have been baptized in Whitchurch on 13th January 1752 and lived in St. Mary's Street. He became a surgeon, although there is no record of his professional qualifications or ability. A quiet, rather stout man, he was a

martyr to the gout and, according to the Whitchurch Parish Register, died on 10th April 1810 having fathered 13 children. His eldest son, William Wycherley Brookes, who died in 1847, was great grandfather to the late Mr. Harry Richards, well known civic dignitary and benefactor. William Brookes is buried in the path leading up to the porch of St. Alkmund's Church.

The census of 1871 revealed that Dr. John Brown, then aged 51, was qualified L.R.C.S. from Edinburgh. He lived originally in St. Mary's Street but moved in 1870 to 19 Dodington. Dr. Molly McCarter informed me that some of the panelling there had been brought from his old house. His household consisted of his wife, three sons, two daughters, a governess, a cook, a housemaid and a groom. Dr. Brown was also family physician to Sir Edward German when he was a small boy in Whitchurch.

Dr. Samuel Tayleur Gwynne M.D., lived in St. Mary's House. He gave lectures in first aid and nursing, but locally is best remembered for his account of the bones of Lord John Talbot, 1st Earl of Shrewsbury, when his skeleton was exhumed in the 1870s. St. Alkmund's Church had fallen down in 1711 and as the debris was cleared away the urn containing the heart of Lord Talbot was found. This was restored to its original resting place in the centre of the porch. The recumbent figure of Sir John was also recovered from the ruins and was carefully preserved in the same relative position. In 1874 it was decided to re-open his tomb. At the simple, impressive ceremony, the Earl and Countess of Brownlow entered the church with Captain Reginald Talbot and other relatives. A curtain was drawn across the vestry window, and the gas burners shed a subdued light on the skeleton as the lid of the coffin was removed. The bones of the great warrior were displayed on the vestry table. A surgical description was given of the bones by Dr. Gwynne, attested by John Bromfield, surgeon, in the *Parish Magazine* for that year. There was a fracture of the skull $2^3/4$ inches long and $^5/8$ths of an inch across, evidently caused by a sharp instrument. The bones generally were well developed, obviously belonging to a muscular man.

Inside the oaken case beneath the recumbent figure, was also found the skeleton of a mouse, and on careful examination Lord Talbot's skull it was found that the cranium was full of a fibrous substance. This, on testing, appeared to be a mouse's nest from which three small mummified mice were extracted.

Dr. Gwynne was a member of the Medical Relief Society which was founded in 1838 to provide medical assistance for families who, although they were not paupers, were nevertheless not able to lay anything aside for sickness. A cursory review by the then rector showed about one hundred cases which had been dealt with and they fell into two classes. The out-ticket enabled the patient to visit the doctor for advice over the course of a fortnight, with the provision of all necessary medicine. The in-ticket enabled the same service to be provided in the patient's home. Payment for the out-ticket was 1s and the in-ticket 1s. 6d., or 2s. if in the country. The rector added the fact that patients were at liberty to choose the medical man they preferred.

Dr. Ambrose George is also mentioned in the 1871 census. He was aged 38 and held a degree of L.R.C.P. from Edinburgh and M.R.C.S. from London. His surgery was in St. Mary's Street.

Another doctor mentioned in the Samuel Bagshaw Gazetteer was Dr. Thomas Groom who was on the staff of the Whitchurch Union Workhouse. He was described as a surgeon.

Other 'surgeons' were John Bromfield of Green End, John Swinnerton of New Street and Thomas Marsh of High Street but their qualifications are not known.

6 Whitchurch Cottage Hospital

The Cottage Hospital was opened on 9 October 1886 at 3 p.m. The site was given by Lord Brownlow and the building was designed by Mr. W.E. Mountford, a London architect.

The project had been set on foot two years previously by a small group of local ladies and gentlemen who had formed a committee, Major Lee being the chairman and Mrs. Waugh and Miss M.A. Kent honorary secretaries. Their aims were to:

(1) engage the services of a trained nurse and an assistant nurse,

(2) to erect a building as their home with a few beds for patients, and

(3) to raise a sum of not less than £1,500.

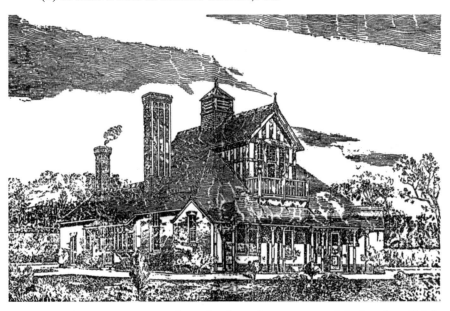

Whitchurch Cottage Hospital on the day of its opening, 9th October 1886, as published in The Herald, *on 16th October*

There was a generous response and the list of donations varied from £100 downwards, resulting in £1,250 being subscribed to the building fund.

To raise the remaining funds they decided to hold a bazaar in the Town Hall. This lasted three days, with many stall holders and generous help from the amateur dramatic performers of the Whitchurch Christy's Minstrels, resulting in the event raising no less than £1,125.

The *Whitchurch Herald* for 16 October 1886 reports:

> The building, though unpretending and inexpensive in character, was arranged and fitted up upon the most modern principles. The design was of great beauty with long tiled gables and wood with plaster walls and panelling. On the ground floor was a male ward with three beds and a female ward of the same number. On the same floor there was an isolation ward with one bed, and a nurses room from which both wards could be observed. There was a verandah on the whole length of the south side of the building and the wards opened out on to it. Lavatories were on the outer corners of both wards. The entrance hall with a rich panelled ceiling opened on to Brownlow Street. Further back there was also a bathroom, operating room and a medical store. A capacious ventilating shaft ran from the inner hall to the roof, terminating in an ornamental turret. Behind the hall was a kitchen, scullery, pantry and other offices. The staircase led from the entrance hall to the upper floor where there was a convalescent ward with a south aspect which opened onto a pleasant balcony. On that floor there were also staff bedrooms. The larder, wash-house, fuel store, mortuary and disinfecting closet were at the back of the hospital.
>
> Speeches were delivered from the verandah. On the opening of the proceedings Major Lee said that, as there was a keen wind blowing he promised that the speeches would be concise. He said he saw the advantage in airy rooms and with skilful medical treatment and kind, ready sympathy, the chances of recovery should be vastly increased. The bazaar had been an immense success. The interest would amount to an estimate of £40 which would raise their total income to £160. Other items would be the Hospital Sunday collection in churches of all denominations, making a possible income not less than £220. In addition to these sums would be payments made by the patients themselves. The amount of payment could vary from 2s. 6d. to 5s. per head.
>
> Dr. Gwynne said that all the medical gentlemen of the neighbour-hood should be invited to become officers of the Institution, and under the care of a sub-committee, which would meet every Monday

morning, would transact general business and for the admission of patients. Patients could be admitted on the recommendation of a doctor supported by a subscriber to a certain amount. Those who could not afford to pay could be attended gratuitously, but in the case of patients paying more than 5s. a week, the Medical Officer of the week should have the privilege, if he should choose, to avail himself of making a reasonable charge on the patient.

Dr. George then spoke particularly about nursing. He felt that this was one of the major social reforms of this century and said he felt that it was only since the Crimean War and Miss Florence Nightingale that we now had Cottage Hospitals in nearly every large town. It was a matter of surprise to him that Whitchurch, which on the map was a centre of an area of 20 miles, had been so long without one.

A brief service was then led by the Rev. W.H. Egerton and Lord Kenyon declared the hospital open and asked all present to partake of tea in the hospital.

The following year, in December 1887, Rev. Egerton reported on Hospital Sunday in the *Parish Magazine* as follows:

No Institution commends itself more strongly to the highest impulse of nature and the fervent exercise of Christian love than the Cottage Hospital in our town.

The hospital was enlarged in 1897 to commemorate Queen Victoria's Diamond Jubilee. It received a modern operating theatre in 1902 and its first x-ray unit in 1904. During the Great War no less than 335 soldiers passed through the hospital.

COTTAGE HOSPITAL.

A NNUAL RUMMAGE SALE will be held on WEDNESDAY, May 2nd, 1906.

The Committee will be glad to receive contributions of Articles at any time.

HUGH BOOTH LEE,
Solicitor, Whitchurch,
Hon. Sec.

WHITCHURCH.

COTTAGE HOSPITAL.—Surgeon for the month Dr. C. H. Gwynn; number of patients in Hospital last week, 12; admitted, 4; discharged, 2; died, 0; remaining in Hospital, 14. Number of Dispensary tickets issued since 30th September, 113. Out-nursing :—Visits, 488; dressings, 677. The Committee gratefully acknowledge the following donations in kind :—Mrs Elliott (Chester) *Graphic*; Mrs Etches, old linen.

One of the monthly reports printed in The Herald *showing the surgeon for the month, and other information*

In the First World War, Prees Heath Camp, just outside Whitchurch, became very well known as a staging post for battalions from the North of England, Scotland and Dublin. My wife's father, who was with the Lancashire Fusiliers, remembered it well. Sadly, many of the young soldiers never returned to their homes. At its height there were about 10,000 troops in the camp. The hospital on the camp was built of brick and contained 500 beds. There were nine main wings, each served by a covered pathway. The hospital can be seen on the photograph.

In 1915 the V.A.D. (Voluntary Aid Detachment) Hospital was opened under General Buston and Mrs. Lambert in the house of Mr. H.L. Storey at Broughall Cottage, Broughall. They had beds for 20 patients and two

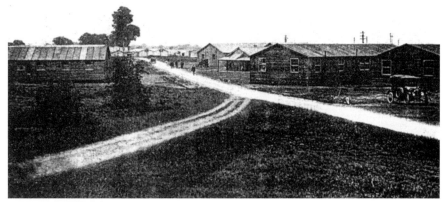

The Military Hospital, Prees Heath, Wartime Postcard of 1915

trained nurses to look after soldiers home from the front. Monetary donations and gifts of food and cigarettes were regularly featured in the *Herald*.

During April 1918 a branch of the organisation 'Comrades of the Great War' was started in Whitchurch, its first Captain being Major Lambert, D.S.O. The Comrades' pledge was 'to work for the moral and social welfare of discharged sailors and soldiers and the dependents of those comrades who had fallen'; it was the forerunner of the British Legion. Membership of the Comrades was 1s.

During the Second World War there was an airfield on Prees Heath and a small hospital was set up in a house overlooking it. Miss Lambert, daughter of Major Lambert, was commandant.

Lloyd George's Social Security Scheme began in 1920. This enabled the ordinary working man and his family to receive medical treatment from a 'panel doctor' and many similar schemes were introduced for factory firms and other groups of workers. When I came into practice they were still using the Lloyd George envelopes to hold notes. Keeping notes in these folders and extracting the relevant ones at the appropriate time was a task for all doctors under the new National Health Service of 1949. The advent of computerised records did have some advantages.

In 1937, as a posthumous gift from Sir Edward German, it was decided to provide a new operating table and to modernize the x-ray equipment, the

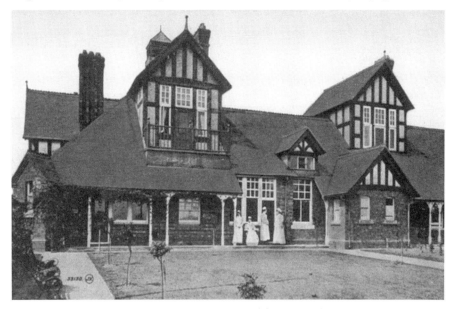

Whitchurch Cottage Hospital between the Wars

49

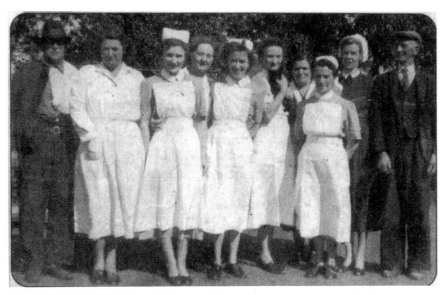

*Staff at Whitchurch Hospital between the wars. On the left is
Thomas Nicholson, one of the gardeners; another gardener is on the left.
Nurse Cadman is third from the right*

whole costing £400. X-rays were, in fact, taken by a nurse, as this was before the days of radiographers in a small hospital. Many will remember Nurse Cadman, for this was her speciality.

When I visited Ruth Wheeler, cook to the Cottage Hospital for many years, she gave me a wonderful account of 'The Cottage' before and in the early days of the Health Service. This is an account in her own words. I am also very indebted to her for many of the good photographs of the old days.

My memories of Whitchurch Cottage Hospital began 57 years ago in April 1946 when I started work as cook, after returning from the ATS as cook in the Army for five years.

The Matron was Miss Edna Evans. She and two sisters and three nurses were the resident nursing staff. Three Red Cross Nurses (non-resident)—Mrs. Cadman, Miss Winsome Lambert and Miss Lowther—were voluntary helpers on the wards. They had all previously nursed the wounded at the Red Cross Hospital at Ash Corner, which closed when the war finished. Mrs. Cadman later joined the staff of the Cottage Hospital and stayed until she retired in the 1970s. Domestic staff consisted of one ward maid and two part-time cleaners.

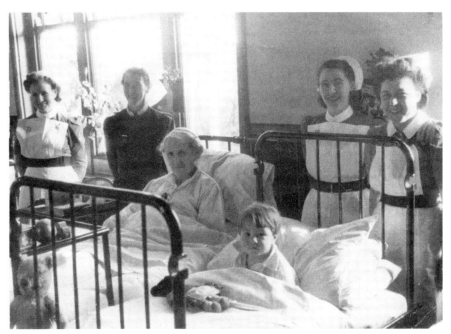

Female Ward Christmas in 1946 when they still had an occasional child patient. The photograph shows, from left to right: Sister Teresa Beddow, Matron Edna Evans, Sister Richards, and Nurse Dyke. The child patient may be Master France

Matron did all the cooking herself for 16 patients and the staff (plus the house keeping). Food was still rationed, so patients brought their Ration Books into hospital when they were admitted, and often their own supply of fresh eggs too. The hospital gardener, Mr. Rogers, provided an adequate supply of vegetables from the kitchen garden and fruit was also plentiful as there was a well stocked orchard. Meat and provisions were supplied by the local butchers and grocers of the town.

Being a voluntary hospital it was very well supported. People gave generously to the upkeep. Donations, legacies, proceeds of shows, fetes, carnivals, concerts etc. all provided the finance required. The management was a committee of highly respected local people, including those in business, landowners, clergy and council officials amongst others. The honorary secretary was a local accountant, Mr. South. Finance was his department. He paid the bills and salaries and held the purse. Perhaps there were about 12 members on the committee, I am not sure, including ladies, one being Mrs. Black, wife of Captain Black of Prees Hall. Two other members were Mr.

Sowden and Mr. Axon (council men). The committee met in the board room of the Cottage Hospital (later the x-ray room) once every month to discuss the business. Following the meeting they toured and inspected the whole of the hospital and grounds.

The hospital included a male ward, a female ward, a private ward, a two-bedded semi-private ward, operating theatre, casualty ward, offices, an x-ray room and accommodation Matron and five nurses upstairs. There were two kitchens and a larder. A mortuary was situated in a corner of the grounds and was always referred to as 'Rose Cottage' by all the staff at the request of Matron Evans.

The hospital, being situated by the side of the A41 and A49 meant that many casualties were brought in from traffic accidents at any time of day or night, and dealt with by one of the local doctors on duty. There was an ambulance for the use of the hospital and that was garaged in the Urban Council yard next to the public mortuary (off Rosemary Lane). The driver was Cyril Williams. He was a council carpenter but drove the ambulance whenever needed, accompanied by a driver's mate. Later drivers were Ron Manning, Ken Winwood and Tom Caulcott. All were Urban Council employees. The ambulance was not too comfortable in those days. Patients were kept warm by hot water bottles but this practice was phased out when it was deemed too dangerous—scalding could take place by a burst bottle. So with the new National Health Service came better vehicles, and later a new Ambulance Station with its own staff.

At Whitchurch Cottage Hospital young people wanting to be nurses were being accepted as probationers for short periods until they found training hospitals that would take them. Changes with the regular staff were also taking place. Nurse Ethel Chester came from her training in Manchester. She was a very popular nurse and worked at the Cottage Hospital throughout until she retired in the late 1970s. Mrs. Cadman stayed and joined the staff mostly doing the x-rays and general nursing. She also retired in the late 1970s.

Boxing Day 1946 began a very severe winter. From then until 6th March snow fell and froze every day. The whole country was blocked. Ambulances were unable to reach patients. Burials could not take place as the ground was too frozen to dig the graves. Here at Whitchurch doctors were doing their rounds on foot. In the wards coal fires were lit and kept in day and night until the thaw came in March. But after the thaw and floods came a beautiful summer. The topic of conversation then was the coming of the National Health Service.

Sister Bromley joined the staff on 26th December 1947. She had returned from the war during which she had served in Queen Alexandra's Imperial Nursing Service in Egypt and Italy. She had nursed the wounded in the field hospitals along with her friend, Miss E. Blackmore, who later joined the Cottage Hospital staff as Matron.

Sister Bromley was offered the Matron's post at Whitchurch Cottage Hospital and remained as Matron until 1957 when she left to marry Mr. Harry Worrall, a solicitor in the town. While Sister Bromley worked on the wards she realised the need for a day room for patients.

Miss Blackmore took over as Matron in 1957, remaining in post until 1977 when she retired after 20 years at the hospital. During the war she had been mentioned in dispatches for bravery under enemy fire, and then trained as a midwife and worked in Leeds, Brighton and Whitchurch before taking the post of Matron at Whitchurch Cottage Hospital, thus following her friend.

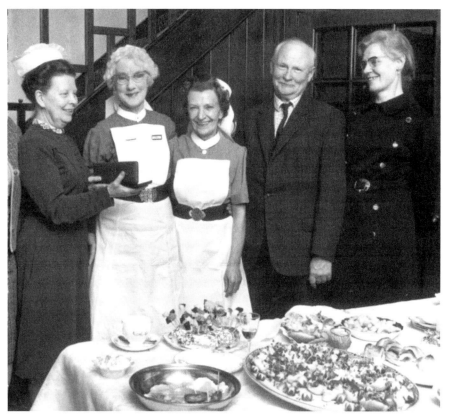

This photograph was taken in the hall of the Cottage Hospital on the occasion of Nurse Chester's retirement party. From left to right: Matron Blackmore, Nurse Chester, Nurse Cadman, Dr. Levingston and Mrs. Worrall

The Cottage Hospital was merged with the adjoining Deermoss Hospital in 1949 when Mr. Wylie was appointed manager of the two hospitals. Then came Mrs. Hutton, Mrs. Casbolt and Matron Blackmore.

I remember some particular incidents during my years at Whitchurch Cottage Hospital. For example, the strong smell of ether filling the air every Tuesday morning in preparation for the operations. The dispensary was adjacent to the kitchen.

Then people regularly brought in sacks of silver paper to be sent away for recycling, for which the hospital received money.

In the 1950s a new Welfare Centre was built in the grounds of the hospital to replace the old clinic at 27 St. Mary's Street, which was a terraced house used as school clinic, chest, orthopaedic and dental clinics and maternity clinic. Mrs. Lawrence, the Health Visitor, occupied the top floor and the ground floor was divided into the various offices and a consulting room, while in a building at the back of the house the orthopaedic nurses and doctors came to do plasters on legs and arms. The orthopaedic people were from Oswestry and visited once a month.

The school clinic was attended to by the District Nurse, usually before school time, every morning. The District Nurse in those days was Miss Rose Evans, who was well known around the town. She visited patients at home and dressed or treated their ailments as directed by the doctors. Most householders paid a monthly subscription of one shilling to enable them, and their families, to call the District Nurse if needed. When off duty Nurse Evans would help in all kinds of charity work. She would tell a fortune (by reading the tea leaves) at a fete or party, for a donation of one shilling to charity.

During the 1960s the League of Friends was formed to raise money for anything required for patients' comfort. Since then the friends have raised thousands of pounds to buy special equipment for the hospital.

Miss Blackmore is now President of the Friends and regularly attends the meetings,at the age of 89.

7   The Coming of the National Health Service

My father once wrote to me as a medical student at Sheffield University to express his views on 'someone called Aneurin Bevan' who was set to alter the arrangements for health provision in the country.

When I arrived in the practice in 1954, having completed National Service as a captain in the RAMC in Germany, the National Health Service had settled down, more or less. No longer did Mr. South do the hospital accounts. We did not have to worry about food, drugs or pay and, as Ruth Wheeler, said, we now had a posh ambulance. General Practitioners were now paid for attending to their 16 patients at the Cottage Hospital and there was a rota for coming in to treat casualties.

My father, Mr. E.S. Clayton, F.R.C.S., M.D., known to the staff as 'the Prof', arrived in Whitchurch in 1942 having come from the position of Medical Superintendent of a very large hospital in Walsall in the Black Country. In the war years he was carrying out 300 operations a year. As Whitchurch was an isolated spot, 22 miles from Shrewsbury Hospital, many of the GPs around used him for consultations. He was also qualified for orthopaedics, including setting fractures and treating quite severe road accidents. At that time several main roads ran right past the door of the Cottage Hospital.

As a boy of 16 I well remember the day when an American army jeep crashed into the corner of our house and ended up in the waiting room in a shower of bricks. The big, tall sergeant said 'Call me Lofty' and father took him into the surgery to treat his few cuts and scratches. The American army got a local builder to repair the hole in our waiting room wall within 48 hours. As Lofty said, 'We are in a hurry'. It was later understood that the convoy was going from Liverpool to the south coast for D Day.

My father's surgical experience was enormous, particularly with regard to emergency surgery. This he performed with relish and great success, doing appendices and strangulated hernia and perforations at all hours of the day and night. On one occasion he was called from playing his cello in the Operatic Orchestra to do an operation and returned again before the end of the performance. On the day he retired he went to Old Trafford to watch cricket, his other great interest. On his death in 1965, in the same week as Winston Churchill died, the whole town was in mourning and on the day of the funeral all the shops in the High Street were closed and St. Alkmund's Church, which then had galleries, was full to capacity. For all his services to the community he received an OBE and when the new day room at the Cottage Hospital was opened it was dedicated to his memory. The plaque, which is now in the foyer of the Whitchurch Community Hospital reads:

THIS TABLET COMMEMORATES THE GIFT TO THIS HOSPITAL OF A NEW OPERATING TABLE AND X-RAY APPARATUS. IN MEMORY OF SIR EDWARD GERMAN FOR THE BENEFIT OF SUFFERERS IN HIS NATIVE TOWN 1937

This tablet commemorates the devoted work of Mr. Edgar Sunderland Clayton F.R.C.S., Surgeon to this hospital from 1942–1965

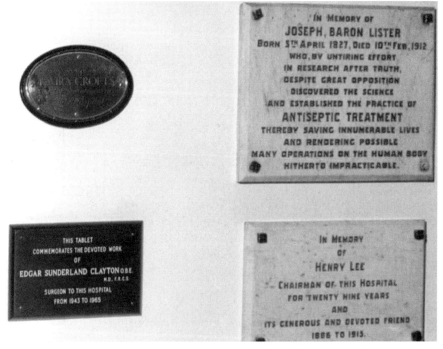

A variety of commemorative tablets preserved in the hospital

'The Cottage' has seen some dedicated surgeons. Mr. Datnow was a gynaecologist from Liverpool. During the war he had a house near to Malpas and used to come into the hospital most saturdays to do an operating list. Gynaecology was nobly kept going after Mr. Datnow by Mr. Sam Burke who came over from Crosshouses Hospital. He was followed by Mr. Alan Blunt who came to Shrewsbury from a post in Queensland, Australia. He kept the operating tradition going until the hospital moved to its new site in 1990.

Other surgeons were Mr. Owen, the Ear, Nose and Throat man who had a marvellous personality. One of his claims to fame was when the hospital invested in smoke alarms. He was smoking his usual pipe in Matron's office when it activated the alarm system and water cascaded down. Another character was Mr. Russell-Johnson, who, at the request of the hospital authorities in Shrewsbury, attended the Whitchurch hospital each month to provide pastoral care for my father's operating and to do an outpatient session. He also partook of tea in Matron's office, consisting of sandwiches and several kinds of cakes served on a tiered cake stand. These always included 'fly pie', a favourite of his, which Mrs. Ruth Wheeler, cook to the hospital for many years, always produced for him. Many other physicians from Shrewsbury attended the hospital to do domiciliary visits at the GP's request.

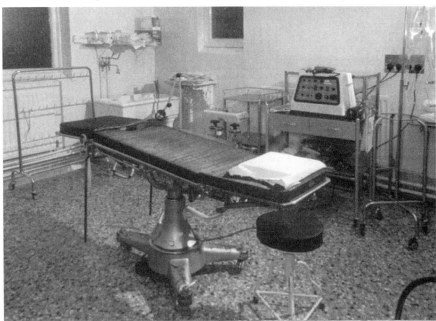

Operating table at the Cottage Hospital

Anaesthetics were given for my father by Dr. Levingston and Dr. Rogerson particularly, and for many years Dr. Giles became the regular anaesthetist for the gynaecological sessions.

Matrons were Mrs. Worrall, followed by Miss Blackmore for many years. Matron Blackmore was a capable and very popular administrator. She lived over 'the shop' in a small flat above the wards and was available day and night to help her staff. She particularly enjoyed my father's operating sessions and she herself was a real 'hands on' performer who liked nothing better than to sit in a comfortable chair and do a difficult suturing of an accident case. I spoke to Matron, who is now 89, and she said these were the best years of her life and she still takes an active interest in The Friends of Whitchurch Hospitals, pushing the trolley around the wards once a week, with her walking stick at the ready. She distributes books and confectionery and 'general advice' as President of the League of Friends. Incidentally, The Friends of Whitchurch Hospitals was launched in 1967. Mrs. Margaret Hiles has been the chairman for quite a number of years, and it is still responsible for raising significant sums of money through donations from people who have been in the hospital. They hold many social events, arrange religious services and a hospital fete every summer. Through their continued efforts, The Friends have provided all manner of equipment for the wards and special departments, such as physiotherapy. They have raised the finance for supplying vehicles for the Shropdoc service based at the Whitchurch Community Hospital which attends out of hours emergencies, on request, throughout north Shropshire, with a doctor in attendance.

An outpatient clinic was built on the car park at the back of the Cottage Hospital in about 1963. Of the consultant medical staff, Dr. Boardman was the first to hold a regular medical clinic, at which he also interpreted the electrocardiograms (tests for heart function). The hospital was fortunate to have the services of Mrs. Garratt, a local resident who was an E.C.G. technician at the Chester Hospital, and regularly came to take these tests. Dr. West ran a diabetic clinic with his own diabetic nurse in attendance. There had been chest physicians attending both the Cottage and Deermoss Hospitals dating from the days when tuberculosis was such a problem.

The nearness of The Robert Jones & Agnes Hunt Orthopaedic Hospital at Oswestry ensured that a large monthly clinic, which was held initially at Deermoss Hospital, was transferred to the new clinic. The consultant brought his own skilled staff and was able to handle problems like renewing plasters and the supervision of artificial limbs. Two names

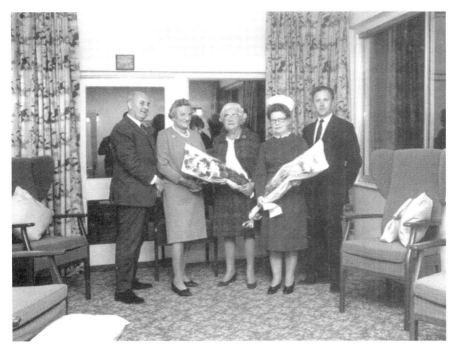

Opening of the Cottage Hospital Day Room.
From left to right: Mr. Frank Leath, Mrs. M. Lee, Mrs. Edgar Clayton
(my mother), Matron Blackmore and Mr. Hough

which stand out in my mind are Mr. McSweeney and, later on, Mr. O'Driscoll. Psychiatric clinics have also been a regular feature for many years with the consultant from Shelton doing domiciliary visits at the request of local GPs.

Many will remember the staff, health visitors and the clinics for ante-natal, child care and family planning. Other midwives and nurses from the old days were Nurse Porter in Prees and Nurse Martin in Ash. There was also a small private maternity unit in Dodington run by Sisters Locker and Lloyd. They were very strict in insisting on two weeks bed rest which gave mothers with large families a chance to have a good rest.

When I came to Deermoss Hospital as hospital practitioner in 1954, the administrator was Mr. Wilson and his wife was the matron. Mr. Birch was the only office employee. There were 101 beds, and I watched patients being taken on stretchers up two flights of very narrow stairs for every admission and we were all pleased when a lift was installed. This was the first of many improvements, including a physiotherapy department which

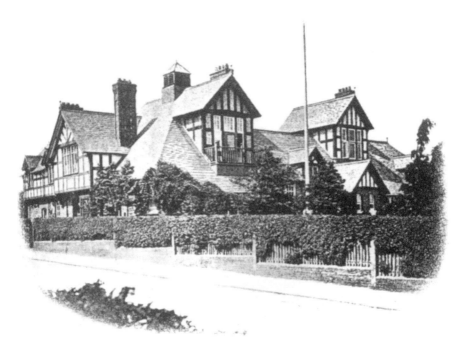

The Cottage Hospital from the roadside

was opened in the old chapel. Some people may remember the physiotherapists—Mrs. Jones, Mrs. Betty Hilton and Mrs. Olwen Dickenson amongst others. Day rooms were opened by enclosing the two balconies and we also started occupational therapy.

In Deermoss Hospital there were really very few relics of the old Poor Law days. We did occasionally still have tramps, especially in the winter time, some of whom had nowhere else to go. They were only supposed to stay two days, but some of them were very ill and remained much longer. I remember one gentleman with a snow-white beard who the nurses called Father Christmas. One year he came to the hospital and a junior nurse shaved off all his whiskers. He turned out to be a young, handsome man. He never came back to us again.

I visited the hospital every morning after my own surgery for many years and returned later in the day to see any emergency cases or new admissions.

A new profession called geriatrics was now coined through the NHS because it was believed that the elderly were not getting a fair deal. The consultants attended the hospital weekly but I was in charge between their visits and could they telephone me for advice. The first geriatric consultant was

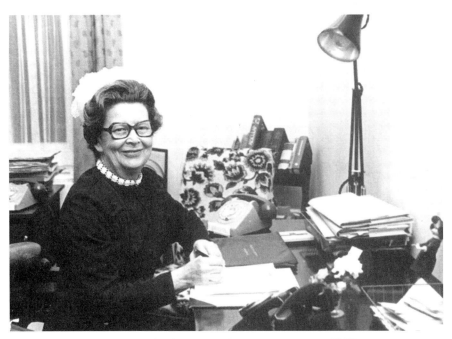

Matron Blackmore on her retirement in 1977

Dr. Irwin. In the 1970s came Dr. Bane. He was from South Africa, from the same university as Christian Barnard, whom he knew. The next consultant in my time was Dr. Khan, who came originally from near Delhi, India. He was very interested in the treatment and the long-term outlook for the elderly patients in his care. He told me that in India, elderly relatives were looked after by their families as a matter of course. With the hospital's rehabilitation facilities his aim was to get as many patients as possible back into their own homes, or when not fit enough, help to arrange for them to go into residential care.

Some patients were admitted from the geriatric bed bureau in Shrewsbury. They were transferred from the medical, surgical and orthopaedic wards for rehabilitation. We also admitted many elderly patients from Whitchurch practices for assessment and treatment within the hospital's competence. We were able to use the x-ray facilities and the link with Shrewsbury for pathology investigations. For social admissions we had a system we called 'family relief' where people could be admitted for a fixed period, normally two weeks, in order to give their carers a rest. Some of our patients were heavily dependant long-stay, including some terminal cases. We closed some beds, leaving two female wards with 26 beds each and a male ward with 20 beds. By the 1970s we had a further wing at the hospital on the ground floor which was a combined day room and dining facility, plus a hairdressing salon.

In the 1970s the nursing staff consisted of seven sisters, five staff nurses, seven SRNs and 41 nursing auxiliaries. During the 33 years that I worked at Deermoss I knew many wonderful members of staff who were loyal, hardworking, totally reliable and with a good ability for preserving their

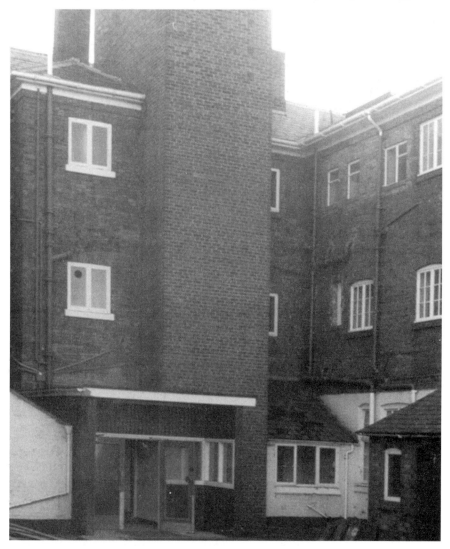

Entrance to Deermoss Hospital showing the lift shaft

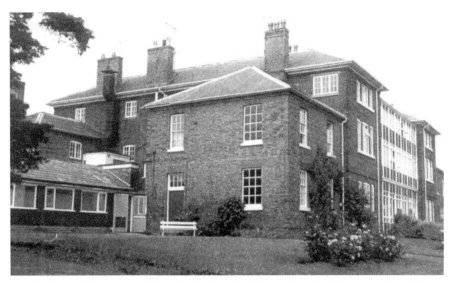

View of Deermoss Hospital after the balconies had been enclosed

sense of humour under, sometimes, very stressful conditions. I could not possibly mention them all individually, although I have never forgotten them and the help that they gave me.

During those years all the staff had a great time at Christmas, when the doctors sang carols on Christmas Eve on the wards and carved the turkeys

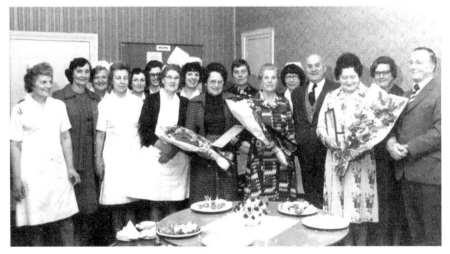

Staff of Deermoss Hospital at Nurse Platt's Retirement Party, with Mr. Leath and Mr. Wylie, nest to whom is Betty Sandells who has supplied many of the photographs in this chapter and the colour section

on Christmas Day. We had annual dances and one of these was held in the Civic Centre when carol singers and the Whitchurch Town Band came into the dance hall.

For the care of elderly patients Deermoss received admissions from all over Shropshire and built up a good reputation for rehabilitation. To replace it Whitchurch now has five Homes for the Elderly.

8   Whitchurch Community Hospital

In July 1977, the Matron, Miss Blackmore, opened the hospital's Annual Garden Fete. In her reassuring address she said 'Our Cottage Hospital recently had much controversial publicity, and while it is only fair to say the statements regarding the building are true, with a will, one can nurse in a tent with a primus stove with a little skill and tender loving care'. She said she thought there would always be a hospital in the town whether on the Cottage Hospital site or another. She also announced that the new unit at Deermoss had been completed and said the hospital had been reborn and would have a tradition to carry on.

In 1990 the two hospitals were joined on the original Deermoss site. At the official opening on 12th October 1990, the Honourable Lloyd Tyrell-Kenyon unveiled a plaque. His ancestor, Lord Kenyon, had opened the Cottage Hospital on 9th October 1886.

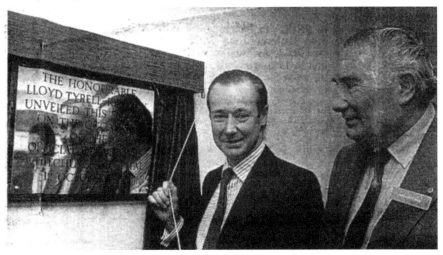

Official opening of the Whitchurch Community Hospital,
watched by Mr. David Lloyd, Chairman of the Shropshire Health Authority

Most of the upper floor of Deermoss was demolished, retaining only some offices, the kitchen and porters' lodge. One of the porters discovered a truncheon; this was clearly used in the Poor Law days when there were vagrants and other doubtful characters about. It is now housed in the Police Museum in Shrewsbury.

All the facilities of both hospitals were retained with the space enlarged and modernized. The only loss was the operating theatre at 'The Cottage'. In the new hospital a small room next to the Accident and Emergency Department was set up with a theatre table for resuscitation purposes and for GPs to do minor operations.

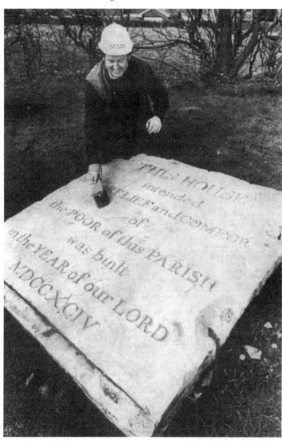

This weighty piece of history was found by Nick Brookfield. It came from the roof of Deermoss Hospital and is now positioned at the entrance to the new Community Hospital

The present hospital is run by the Shropshire Primary Care Trust. There are 38 beds for rehabilitation and on Beech Ward 16 beds for the elderly mentally infirm (E.M.I.). There is a minor injury unit and facilities for 'Shropdoc'. There are clinics for the visiting consultants and a wide range of nursing clinics. Physiotherapy and occupational therapy areas have also been expanded, offering a local service to the community as well as the hospital and is staffed by qualified physiotherapists and occupational therapists.

Adjoining the hospital is the Bradbury Day Centre which is run by Social Services and has facilities for elderly people. They can be collected by transport from home and have the use of the centre, including lunch and the hydrotherapy pool.

The old hospital chapel is now a Healthy Living Centre providing a coffee bar and space for patients and their visitors to meet. It also organizes lectures and advisory groups on topics such as blood pressure, obesity, diabetes and other life threatening conditions, in a friendly atmosphere.

All the medical practitioners in the town attended on the Cottage Hospital and have always worked closely together. Medical care out of regular hours is now provided by a combined organization of doctors over a wide area called 'Shropdoc' based at Whitchurch Community Hospital.

Doctors' Practices in the town
At Dr. McCarter's Practice, in Dodington, one of the earliest doctors was Dr. Brown who has already been mentioned in connection with the census of 1877. He lived in St. Mary's House initially and then moved to Dodington. Dr. Edward Arthur Perram is mentioned in Kelly's Directory of 1909 as a factory surgeon, presumably at Smith's Foundry. Another doctor at the practice was Dr. Anderson and many people will remember Drs. James and Molly McCarter. They retired in 1973, Dr. Molly McCarter living in part of the surgery house until her death in 2001.

At the Dodington Surgery in 1886 there was Dr. George who was known to be at the opening ceremony of the Cottage Hospital on 9th October that year. Dr. Arthur Muriel Watkins and his brother Dr. Vincent Watkins took over in about 1900. Dr. Arthur, as well as being a GP, was medical officer to the Whitchurch Union Workhouse. He delivered many notable characters including a well known local historian. Dr. Clough ran the practice before the last war, until my father appeared in 1942. I joined my father in 1954. He died in 1965 and some ten years later Dr. Paul Wilson joined the practice. When I retired, my daughter Ruth Clayton took my place thereby making three continuous Clayton generations. Dr. Andrew Rogers has now joined the practice.

The Richmond House Surgery was formerly at Bark Hill House. Dr. Lee-Abott, a retired army Colonel, arrived at Bark Hill House in 1909. Dr. Rogerson arrived in 1939 but immediately left to take up duties as a naval officer in the Second World War. In his absence the practice was run by his wife and her sister, Mrs. Wright, who were both medically qualified. The surgery is now run by Drs. Terry and Teather.

The Bridgewater Surgery started with Dr. Levingston in about 1920 and his nephew, Dr. Flewett, joined the practice at the same time as I did the

Dodington Surgery, after our National Service. Dr. Giles joined Dr. Flewett and the practice is now in the hands of Dr. Thompson and Dr. Snelling.

The Future

Huge advances have been made in all kinds of medical and surgical techniques, helped in many cases by the needs of two world wars. Antibiotics arrived in the Second World War and their limitations are only now becoming more apparent. At the beginning of the 21st century surgeons are now operating through keyholes and transplanting many organs. We now have birth control made possible by the Pill and better treatment of cancer and some other diseases. However, the changes in family values have imposed many problems in people's approach to health care, not only with stress-related illnesses but many social problems.

Whitchurch people appreciate the many new facilities for diagnosis and treatment, as well as having their relatives and friends near to them, avoiding long trips to Shrewsbury and Telford hospitals. On speaking to patients in the hospital who have been transferred from other busy district hospitals for rehabilitation, they comment on the quietness, good food, informal atmosphere and the general cleanliness and tidiness of the hospital; 'rather like home'. In Whitchurch the emphasis has always been on rehabilitation, doing everything possible to return patients to their own homes in the community.

If the Revd. Francis Egerton, one of Shropshire's eccentrics and one who played an important role in setting up the House of Industry, could see what is available to us in Whitchurch today, he would undoubtedly be well pleased.

Sources

Chapter 1 Early Medical Care
Cambridge History of Medicine, edited by Roy Porter
Mediolanum, Excavations at Whitchurch 1965–6, by G.D.B. Jones

Chapter 2 Medicine in Britain
Accounts of the Talbot Household 1394–1425, by Barbara Ross
Plague at Whitchurch, by J.F.D. Shrewsbury
Pepys' Diary - The Shorter Pepys, by Robert Latham
An Inquiry into the Cause and Effects of Variolae Vaccinae, a disease
discovered in some of the Western Counties of England, particularly
Gloucestershire and known by the name of Cowpox, by E. Jenner (London, Sampson Low,
      1798)
The Greatest Benefit to Mankind, by Roy Porter
Eminent Doctors, 1885, by G.P. Bettany

Chapter 3 John Tylston and other Whitchurch Doctors
The Complete Works of Matthew Henry, Baker Books, USA
Eighteenth-century Medics, 1985, by P.J. Wallis, R.V. Wallis and T.D. Whittet, PHIBB
The Journeys of Celia Fiennes
University of Keele, Shropshire Historical Documents, ed. Alannah Tomkins
Medical Register of 1783, Wellcome Institute

Chapter 4 Deermoss Hospital — The House of Industry
The Rector's Book at St. Alkmund's Church, Whitchurch, much of which is in Francis
      Egerton's own handwriting
The late Mr. R.B. James looked at the Account Books for the House of Industry between
      1795-1805
Poor Law Union Records, SRRC
The Bridgewater Millions, 1942, by Bernard Falk
A History of Prees, by Mary Preston
Prees Vestry Accounts, courtesy of Mrs. Blower
Whitchurch Herald

Chapter 5 Victorian England
Bagshaw's *Directory* of 1851
Census of 1871

Chapter 6 Whitchurch Cottage Hospital
Whitchurch Herald 1869 and 1886
Papers from the Revd. W.H. Egerton, Rector of St. Alkmund's Church

Index

Numbers in italics refer to illustrations and *CS* to the colour section

Frank 'n' Stan's Bucket List
#1: TT Races

ISBN-13: 978-1985302136

ISBN-10: 1985302136

First printing, March 2018

Cover artwork by Paul Nugent

Proofreading, editing, formatting, and design provided by Dave Scott and Cupboardy Wordsmithing

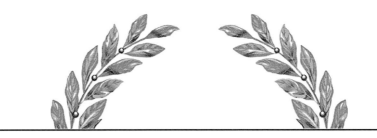

Frank 'n' Stan's Bucket List
#1: TT Races

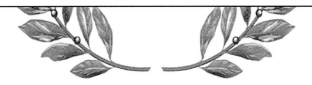

J C Williams

Other Books
by

J C Williams

*Cabbage Von Dagel: An action-packed
wartime spy and detective thriller*

*Hamish McScabbard: A Viking action and
adventure story*

The Flip of a Coin

*The Lonely Heart Attack Club: The perfect
laugh-out-loud romantic comedy
(The Lonely Heart Attack Club Book 1)*

*The Lonely Heart Attack Club
'Wrinkly Olympics'
(The Lonely Heart Attack Club Book 2)*

The Seaside Detective Agency

table of contents

Dedicated to the heroes, on and off the track, who make The Isle of Man TT the greatest sporting spectacle in the world.

Dave Quirk, the epitome of back-of-the-van racing — your assistance has been invaluable.

chapter one

"Can I phone someone for you, Mr Cryer?" asked the petite receptionist. She was pretty and gave him a look of compassion that was genuine, not forced. She held her gaze, tilting her head as she curled her lips, revealing a faint smile that brought a glimmer to her vibrant blue eyes.

Frank stared vacantly in her direction. He could hear the words and see her lips moving, but it didn't compute.

"How about your wife or children? Do you have children?"

He took a step forward. "Could you get me a glass of water, Miss?"

She smiled and moved toward the water dispenser located next to the vast oak reception desk. "You should let me phone someone," she said, handing him the fragile plastic cup.

He felt like he was in a dream sequence, expecting to wake up any moment. He drained the contents of the cup and looked at the people sat patiently in the sterile waiting room. The incessant ringing from behind the reception desk reverberated through his skull like a pneumatic drill. The faces that looked back at him from the waiting room appeared to melt in front of his eyes.

He felt like the room was spinning around him, as if on an acid-fuelled adventure, before the firm vibration in his trouser pocket roused him back to reality.

"Yes, hello, Molly," he said, before listening for a moment. And then, "I'm sorry, I forgot." He raised his hand to his forehead. "I know I said I'd be there, but... look, I'm sorry. Did your mum not make it either?"

Frank nodded his head as the voice on the other end became louder and more heated. He rolled his eyes as he moved to one side to allow an elderly lady to collect a prescription slip.

"Look, I'm sorry, there's nothing more I can say," he insisted. The frustration in his face intensified. "What's so important that I'd miss you coming out of hospital?" he said, mirroring the caller's words. *"What's so important?"* he repeated, with controlled aggression in his breaking voice.

Frank looked around at his current surrounding and took comfort from the friendly receptionist looking back at him — maybe she was a nurse and not a receptionist, he thought.

"Molly, it's not always about you, you know," he said, returning his attention to his phone. "You're like your mother at times. Selfish!"

He listened for a moment longer as he pressed his palm down on the desk, "Me, I'm... I've... I'm at a work thing, I'm sorry. I couldn't get out of it."

He gripped the corner of the desk with such force that his knuckles turned white. "I know you've been in hospital and I said I'd be there to see how it turned out, but, as I said, I've got something on that I couldn't reschedule."

He moved the phone an inch away from his head as the volume increased to an extent that it was in danger of rupturing his eardrum. A woman on a rant is a challenge to interrupt so he stood patiently and waited for the opportune moment...

"I'm bloody selfish?" he shouted, now commanding the attention of those seated in the waiting room.

"I'm selfish," he repeated. "I see. Did you forget that it was me working eighteen hours a day that keeps you in your designer clothes and pays for that swanky flat? When was the last time you asked how I was? I know I said I'd be there, but

2

I couldn't make it, and don't forget that it was me that paid for the operation to make your bloody tits bigger, so excuse me for being selfish for once in my life!"

He mashed the keyboard to end the call, before slamming the phone down on the desk. He placed his face in his hands, taking several deep breaths to compose himself. He looked back at the receptionist, who had wheeled herself a couple of extra feet away from him.

"I'm sorry about that," he said, raising his hands in submission. "I've got one, by the way."

"Pardon me?" she said.

"You asked if I had children. I've got one. A girl called Molly. A girl called Molly who by now has an expensive pair of extended knockers. I'm sorry about this, but, you know, it's not been the best of days."

"Take these," she said, moving closer to him.

She handed him a pile of brochures, which he glanced at before placing them inside his jacket pocket.

"If you need anything, just ask," she said.

"Thank you... I mean that, you've been wonderful. And I will. Call you, that is."

Frank turned, offering a conciliatory smile toward the patrons of the waiting room who were all now aware of his daughter's endowments.

The doctor's surgery had motion-sensor glass doors that met each other in the middle. One of them was lazy and operated about half the speed as the other. He'd noticed it on the way in and had made a mental note to remember this on the way out. He was still reeling from the conversation with Molly, however, when he just remembered the thing he was meant to remember — too late — and his face smashed off the glass door that opened slower than it should.

The greasy imprint of his nose was visible on the glass as were several others whose owners had been, it would appear, equally as distracted. Frank smiled as a little girl walking toward the door had observed his misfortune and was now doubled-over laughing as her mother yanked her arm whilst trying to suppress her own laughter.

"I'd watch that door if I were you," said Frank to the little girl — who now had mirthful tears running down her cheeks — ruffling her hair as she passed by with her mum. "It's a magnet for proboscis prints, you know."

He was grateful for the distraction, despite the pain of his throbbing beak, and took a deep breath of the air — which was bracing for a March morning. His phone was buzzing again in his pocket, but he chose to ignore it, reasoning it would be another tirade.

It was a little after 10 a.m. but the morning rush hour had not abated. Frank stepped between two parked cars and recoiled as a white-van man passed him at speed, sounding his horn as he extended his middle finger to further convey his fond regards.

Frank resisted the temptation to return the gesture, and he crossed the road with greater attention. His Mercedes taxi was parked in the corner of the pay-and-display car park; he was fortunate to find a space at that time of the morning.

His pace quickened as he caught sight of a pencil-thin parking attendant who looked like he was wearing his dad's trousers, stood looking at the sticker on his car.

"Hello, sir, hello!" shouted Frank as he broke into a gentle trot. "I'm here, come on, I'm only five minutes late."

The attendant — Terry, according to his name badge — greeted him with a warm smile, which was somewhat unnerving in view of the circumstance.

Terry looked over the rim of his wire glasses which sat on an impressive Roman nose, and then flicked his arm smartly forwards to reveal his watch. "That's OK, sir," he said, tilting his head slightly. "I thought I'd wait here for five minutes before issuing a ticket. I often find, in this job, that people are never more than five minutes late. And by being patient for a moment or two longer, we get happy customers who'll come back and use us again."

Frank was taken off-guard and thought he must be on camera in some bizarre television show. "Thanks, Terry," he said suspiciously, his eyes darting around the car park. When it was clear there was no ulterior motive, and no hidden camera, he smiled and climbed inside his plush car, pulling the sticker off the window. It left a thin ragged remnant that would require a firm fingernail to remove later.

He started his car and observed Terry through the rear-view mirror, stood there continuing his surveillance duties with an endearing smile on his face.

"Terry!" shouted Frank, climbing back out of his car. "Terry, wait there a moment, please!"

Frank jogged forward and offered his hand, which was cautiously received. "Look, what you just did has made my day," explained Frank. "I can afford the ticket and, to be honest, I deserved it. I'm late, after all."

Terry didn't speak but looked at his hand which was enclosed in Frank's for a little longer than was comfortable before finally letting go.

"Terry," Frank continued. "People... see, people getting back to their car is the final aspect of their journey. If they've had a shit day, they know that salvation is available by getting back into the cocoon that is their car and being able to drive away from all the craziness, or whatever has made them have a shit day. If they try to escape and find you putting a ticket on their car, that's why people get irrationally upset."

Terry said nothing, and let Frank go on.

"I mean, it's not your bloody fault that they didn't buy a ticket for the correct amount of time. Like me. I shouldn't have been so stupid, should I? But you just happen to be the final link in the chain of what could be the worst day that person has ever had."

Frank stood at the rear of his car and pushed down on his greying hair that blew erratically in the sharp wind. "Terry, you most likely think I'm mental, or at the very least, unhinged, but you had it in your gift to push me over the edge this morning. But you didn't. I'd have paid my forty-pound fine—"

"Sixty," said Terry reflexively.

"Sixty, then," Frank agreed. "But the point is, I'd have paid that fine, eventually, probably after the third reminder, and I'd have forgotten about you, only left with the bitter memory of the parking ticket. I certainly wouldn't have remembered that your name was Terry. I certainly wouldn't have recalled the distinguished, impressive nose, or the man that was proud to put his high-viz jacket on every morning to survey his castle and restore order where they were none. All I would have remembered was, just when I thought my shit-fuelled day couldn't get any worse, up pops a jumped-up power monger whose sole duty that day was to make my life even more of a misery."

Frank shifted his weight, then continued.

"Terry, you didn't do that. And you didn't have to do what you did. But now, when I think of this horrible day, I'll think of you and how you had it in your power to kick a man when he was down. You didn't do that, Terry. And I genuinely mean it, when I say, *thank you.*"

Terry smiled and took a step forward. He placed his hand on Frank's shoulder and, as appeared to be the theme of the day, tilted his head. "You'll be fine, it's not the end of the road," he said gently as he leaned down to pick up one of the brochures that had fallen from Frank's pocket.

Terry glanced at it for a moment before handing it back to Frank, who illogically now felt a wave of vulnerability.

"My mum had the same thing," continued Terry. "And four years later she's still going strong and always onto me about getting a girlfriend, a house, or even a better job, but I like this job and I wouldn't be any happier if I was stuck in an office, nine-till-five. You need to do what you enjoy."

Frank twisted the brochure between his hands and nodded. "I wish you were around twenty years ago to tell me that."

He paused for a moment before continuing.

"You know what, Terry, I was meant to meet you today. Call it fate, or whatever. But there's a reason I met you. I'm going to go home, just now, and do something to my wife that I should have done six months ago."

"Lucky girl," said Terry.

"No, trust me, if you met her, or at least spoke to her, that's the last thing you'd want to do. She's not a nice person. I'm going to go home and tell the bitch I'm leaving her."

Terry scratched his chin. "Okay... didn't see that one coming."

Frank paced on the spot, clasping his hands together like a church and steeple before him and rubbing the index fingers of the steeple together while placing them against his lips. His pointer fingers grew warm from the friction.

"She knew I was at the doctor's today, but was too busy to come, not that I wanted her to," he said. "She's with her fitness instructor, Boris. A huge blond-haired chap, from Latvia, or that neck of the woods, but it's more the horizontal exercise she's getting, if you know what I mean."

Terry was unsure if he should adopt the sympathetic-looking, tilted-head approach once again. "Are you going to hit him... the instructor, Boris?" he asked.

"Hit him? Good god, no. He's built like a brick shithouse. He'd eat me alive... No, if anything, I should be buying him a pint. He's committed the ultimate sacrifice and should be commended. My wife is horrible, plain and simple. She only married me for my money, I know that. I'm what... sixty-one, and she's fifteen years younger than me, but she's only happy when she's got a credit card in her hand and only smiles when the dentist is bleaching her teeth for the umpteenth time. The sad thing is, my daughter has inherited most of her less-than-endearing features, and those she hadn't, she's now had enlarged. I've been putting this off for months, but, life's too short. Thanks, Terry!" Frank placed both his hands upon Terry's shoulders and met his eyes. "Thank you!" he said again with sincerity.

Frank climbed back into his car and watched as a bemused car-park attendant continued on his rounds.

His phone had continued to vibrate, so he took it reluctantly from his pocket. His trepidation at the call, however, was replaced by a warm smile when he saw several texts from Stan:

> Hiya, Frank. Hope you're well, pal, just checking in to see how it went. Don't rush back, I'll look after things at work x.

It was only a text, but it meant a great deal. In that one message, he'd had more compassion than from his own family. Frank replied:

> 1. Not the best news, but I'm fine, honest. 2. I'm going home to tell her I'm leaving her...

Frank re-read the words and the reality set in. Rather than a feeling of dread, he sat back in the sumptuous leather seat and felt a warmth of contentment spread through him.

Immediately, his phone lit up once again:

> 1. We'll get you through, whatever it is. 2. Good, she's a bitch... Great tits though.

Frank laughed as he put the phone back in his pocket.

He checked his hair in the rear-view mirror which was erratic. He was a youthful sixty-something, and if he dyed his greying hair, he could easily be mistaken for late forties. He still had most of his hair, his teeth were in good shape, and other than a slight paunch — which was fairly easily rectifiable in the gym, if he'd had a mind to rectifying it — he was in good shape. Despite this, his wife was all too eager to point out that he was ready for the knackers' yard, and the more he listened to her the more he started to believe it. Today could easily have been the worst day in his life, but, bizarrely, he was feeling optimistic as he drove out of the car park, giving Terry an enthusiastic thumbs-up for good measure.

Frank had never been particularly materialistic. He could appreciate the finer things in life, of course, but their house — with its tree-lined private driveway leading to a cul-de-sac with five opulent detached mansions — was all her idea.

He never thought of himself as rich; it'd taken many years to build up his business, so wealth accumulation had been a gradual process and, as such, difficult to place a finger on the turning point. That is, there was no one moment when Frank suddenly thought to himself, *"Ah, I'm rich."*

He'd bought his first taxi with Stan when they were eighteen, when most their age would be out drinking. They invested everything they'd made, and one car became two, then five, until eventually they had over one hundred and thirty and were one of the largest operators in Liverpool.

He always felt uncomfortable in the house surrounded by those that were exceedingly materialistic. When they married, Helen had a penchant for a nice meal and an exotic holiday but she was, ultimately, happy with her lot. The house had changed her for the worse; she'd become obsessed with possessions, labels, and what other people thought of her and, more so, what they thought of her husband. For years, she'd insist that Frank leave the taxi on the main road, for instance, and walk into the house. She gave the impression that she was a little embarrassed about him, controlling what he wore and how he should conduct himself in front of people that really didn't matter to their lives.

Her actions hurt him initially, but when he realised she was with him for his wallet he cared a little less each day. He'd park the taxi in front of the house and think nothing of parading around the garden in tight-fitting shorts on a warm summer's day. She was particularly impressed when she came home, on one occasion, to find him and Stan drinking beer in a cheap inflatable swimming pool. The truth is, the neighbours were a decent sort, and fond of Frank. They could see Helen for what she was: mutton dressed up as lamb. The thing that hurt him the most was seeing his little angel turning out more and more like her mother.

He pulled his car up outside his neighbour's house and, to the uninitiated, must have looked very much like a taxi waiting to pick up a fare. He placed both hands firmly on the wheel for a long moment, before finally letting go and taking up the pile of brochures — clutching them tightly as if they gave him a source of strength. He stepped out and walked gingerly past the sprawling lawn toward his own home and stood at the head of the driveway looking at his house. It was impressive, but perhaps too modern for the look it was trying to achieve. He'd never seen Boris's car, but the gaudy-looking BMW with an oversized spoiler, there in the drive, gave him the impression that his wife was currently 'mid-session' on her fitness regime.

Frank tried the door and to his surprise it was unlocked. He wasn't stealthy as he entered his home and for a moment he felt like he was invading on other people's privacy. The polished wooden floorboards did little to cushion his footsteps as he approached the archway to the kitchen. A shrill voice startled him, but it was the radio in the corner that had been left unattended. Two cups of tea sat on the farmhouse kitchen table, still half-full, as if those consuming them had business elsewhere. A door just off the kitchen led to the insulated double garage where his wife — at great expense — had installed a fully equipped gym.

Frank looked at the door for a moment. There were two possible outcomes for the current situation: 1) Boris and his wife were behind the door dressed in Lycra, or 2) The gym was empty, and his wife was upstairs promoting pan-European relationships. He thought he wouldn't care, but as he reached for the polished chrome handle, he knew his life, as he'd known it, could soon change forever.

He didn't want to appear like a typical jealous spouse, so he opened the door gently and casually walked inside. The room was empty, but it was warm, and the smell of fresh sweat hung in the air. Scenario № 2 was now presenting itself as the most likely outcome in his thought process.

A pair of men's trainers and a blue vest with a blackened sweat patch lay on the floor — cast aside as if removed in haste. Frank booted one of the trainers and marched with vigour, through the kitchen and up the winding staircase to the upstairs landing. Rather than dwell, he kicked aside the assortment of underwear outside their bedroom. *"Bitch isn't even trying to be discreet,"* he thought.

As he pushed the door open, his heart smashed through his chest. He'd rehearsed what he'd say when he walked in the room, and it was going to be memorable, poignant, and possibly scathing. Yes, definitely scathing. But as soon as he saw his wife lying naked on the bed, his mind went blank.

He walked forward a couple of paces, but if he was looking for inspiration it was certainly eluding him. They looked at each other, he and his wife, like they were in a Mexican standoff. Helen was like a rabbit caught in the headlights and even though it was her husband she reached for something to cover her expensive, cosmetically-enhanced modesty. She didn't break eye contact and unfortunately for her, however, the first thing she grabbed was a pair of black-leather Y-fronts with an impressive appendage attached...

that started to vibrate expectantly when she thrust it against her chest.

"Are they my undies?" asked Frank sarcastically.

Helen went to speak, though bought a little more time with an awkward cough to clear her throat. It wasn't the sort of cough that was necessary. It was more the sort of cough you give your doctor when he gets hold of your bollocks.

"You're home, Frank? You, em, never come home at this time." Helen cringed as the splashing noise of a running tap came from the en-suite bathroom.

Frank turned from her and waited patiently for the bathroom door to open. Boris eventually appeared, looking manly and rugged. Frank felt instantly pathetic and somewhat emasculated as he looked at the sculptured naked physique stood before him in a state of partial arousal.

Frank had no intention of aggression, but even he was disappointed by his own actions as he reached forward to shake Boris's hand. He was always polite, of course, but on this occasion it was probably ill-timed.

Boris looked Frank in the eye, then over to Helen, and back to Frank.

Boris took a toothbrush from his mouth as a small sliver of paste ran down his chin. "Are you going to hit me?" he asked. "You can have one, but don't go crazy."

Frank turned up his nose in anger, revealing his front teeth but the threat level was, at best, mediocre, with Boris not even moving from his current position. For reasons unknown to him, Frank still had his hand held out in front like he was greeting an old friend. He became aware of how close his hand was to Boris's crotch which was slowly decreasing in mass like an old balloon.

As Boris's manhood descended, Frank's hand rose, turning, as it did, into a tight fist with forefinger firmly extended, and coming to a stop when held in front of the naked lothario's face.

"That's... my... FUCKING... toothbrush," snarled Frank through gritted teeth.

Boris now took a step back. The toothbrush drooped slowly as his jaw relaxed, before breaking free and tumbling down onto the tiled floor — leaving a smear of molten toothpaste as it hit.

Helen, reflexes intact, sprang to attention, sat up in the bed, the still-vibrating dildo clutched tightly against her chest, massaging her heart. Despite the swift, animated motion of her shift in position, her expensive breasts held firm.

"You pathetic sack of shit!" she shouted. "You're more worried about your bloody toothbrush than the naked man about to ravish your wife!" She gripped the leather Y-fronts and flung them toward Frank. The weight of the attached rubber phallus caused them to fly through the air like a missile.

The realistic-looking penis hit Frank directly on the side of the temple with a loud slap. He staggered, putting a hand toward his head before falling onto one knee. As he fell, he reached out to steady himself. He shook his head to clear his senses and became acutely aware that he was now supporting himself by gripping onto Boris's flaccid tallywhacker.

Frank stared at the cock in his hand. "Some things are sacred," he said thoughtfully. "A man's toothbrush is one of those things."

Rather than release his grip, Frank held firm. He used the leverage he had, forcing himself back to a standing position, pushing himself up whilst forcing the other man down. Boris screamed like a fourteen-year-old girl at a concert.

Frank, now back at full height, brushed his hands together briskly with a few quick claps to clean the cock off them, in a motion that might also be interpreted as an *and-that-takes-care-of-that* motion.

"You might have a short wait for your afternoon romp," said Frank laughing, in reference to Boris now curled up on the floor cupping his genitals.

"At least it's worth waiting for!" Helen shouted, like a petulant child.

Frank smiled. "Rather him than me. He deserves a bloody medal putting up with you, you sanctimonious, selfish, greedy cow. And... I know you're a bit stupid, but, in case you hadn't figured it out... I'm leaving you!"

Frank took one final look at Boris before casually marching back out of the door. "Oh, and just so you know," he called over his shoulder, "I've cancelled all of your credit cards. So the only plastic you're left with is the contents of your oversized tits. And, Boris? You can keep the toothbrush. My gift to you. I'll get another."

"Thank you," Boris said weakly, fighting back tears.

"I hope you're both very happy together. All the best!"

Frank slammed the bedroom door behind him and walked across the landing. He looked with disdain at an oversized vase sat proudly on the hall table. He'd never liked it — it was tacky, bought on a whim, by her, to impress her friends. Call it childish, but he stopped and turned on a sixpence. He looked at the vase for a moment and thought of hurling it down the stairs. Instead, he took the gaping mouth of the vase and placed it cautiously over the handle of the bedroom door. He could have smashed it himself, but he gained more satisfaction knowing that she'd smash it herself when she opened the bedroom door.

Frank stomped back to his car and by now the neighbours — who'd obviously heard the commotion — were now pretending to busy themselves in the garden next door.

"Morning, Frank, everything okay with you?" asked George, clearly fishing for information. "Helen not with you?"

George received a firm elbow in his ribs from his equally nosey wife, Susan, as Frank waved in acknowledgement.

"All good, George, thanks. Helen is not with me. Quite right. I've just told her that I'm leaving, so, all in all, a great day. She's upstairs with her lover, Boris... and his friend, Gustav, I think his name was, although he was wearing a rubber mask, so, I may have misheard. It was like a medieval dungeon when I walked in that bedroom — all sorts of harnesses, costumes, and about fifteen dildos lying on the bed. I think one of them was petrol-powered. Susan, you should have a word with Helen, I'm sure she doesn't need to keep all of them for herself — probably make sure you wash them first, though."

A great weight had been lifted and, for the first time in many months, Frank felt happy. He climbed into his car, rejuvenated. He had no idea where he was going to go and had no clothes, or toothbrush, for that matter. But it didn't matter; he was walking out on one sorry chapter in his life and starting a new one. And even if the new one should be cut short, it would at least be happier than the one he'd been currently living.

chapter two

Frank 'n' Stan's taxis were a feature of the city. A small logo of the green mythical creature immortalised in Mary Shelly's novel adorned the side of each car, making them instantly recognisable. Head office was an unassuming office, in a scruffy back alley in the heart of the town centre. To bring order to the operational helm of this empire required a certain temperament: calm under pressure, organised, and able to shepherd the drunken hordes, but, ultimately, the ability to coordinate over one-hundred hairy-arsed, surly taxi drivers.

The dubious honour fell upon the very broad shoulders of Stella. She'd been with the business since Day One and would, at best, be described as an acquired taste. She was a considerable unit, with a prodigious neck that all but absorbed her chin. Her hair was a natural perm, wrapped so tight that it looked and felt like Velcro. She could chastise a tardy driver one moment and, in an instant, turn on the elegant charm to answer the phone which rang incessantly.

For her, the smoking ban was a challenge rather than an edict. Those brave enough to enter her domain were faced with a plume of smoke from her ever-present cigarette curling up into a dense cloud that hung in the air, swirling slowly around her. It moved languidly and yet it raged relentlessly. Like Jupiter's Great Red Spot, it was a storm that had survived for years, as long as anyone could remember, and showed no signs of dissipating or remitting.

Stella sat behind her aged desk. The work counter separating her from others was shoulder-high, ostensibly to prevent drunken, angry patrons from raining abuse upon her, though the unspoken truth of it was more the other way around — that those who might find themselves unfortunate enough to cross her path, rather, should be protected from Stella.

Frank and Stan had an office at the rear of the building with a linked door, but with a separate entrance if they wanted to avoid the congested waiting room.

"Have we heard from Frank yet?" asked Stan, peering from behind the door.

Stella barely moved. She had a fag hanging from her mouth that was more ash than fag. How it remained intact and held in place was quite remarkable.

"I'm his P.A. now?" she asked through pursed lips whilst managing to effortlessly contain the tenuous state of her cigarette in what can only be described as a miracle.

She held her eyes on him for a moment before exhaling an acrid burst of smoke. "Have you dyed your hair?" she asked, looking off the rim of her glasses. Nothing escaped Stella.

Stan withdrew slightly. "What?" he stuttered. "Of course not."

Stella removed the fag, flicking the contents into an overfilling ashtray as she forced herself from her leather chair that had a perfect imprint of her ample bum cheeks.

"Come here," she insisted with her authoritative, gravelly voice.

Stan pushed the door open and reluctantly walked forward. He was the same age as Frank but was struggling to accept the prospect of ageing as well as Frank. His dress sense was twenty years younger than he was, and from a distance his excessive gold jewellery looked like it'd been bought from a market stall — but it was all genuine, if not somewhat ostentatious.

"You've had a spray-tan?" continued Stella. She started to laugh, but it sounded more like the laboured efforts of an old car engine being started.

Stan started to blush, but it was difficult to tell under the generously applied layer of gravy browning. His hair was jet-black, but the giveaway was the perfectly groomed eyebrows that now looked like two manicured black caterpillars. "I've got a date!" he conceded. "I wanted to look my best!"

"I hope you're going to ask for a refund, then," cackled Stella. "And Don Johnson just called — he wants to know when he's getting his suit back?"

"Very droll... So, you've not seen Frank?" repeated Stan.

Stella took a moment, settling first back into her chair before answering.

"No, he had an appointment this morning, but he'd not been back here and he's not turned his radio back on. With all his bloody money, I still don't know why he insists on driving that cab around."

"Probably to get away from you," whispered Stan.

"I bloody heard that, Stan — or should I say, David Hasselhoff."

Stan gave her a wry smile.

"I'm going out for a bit, if you hear from him, tell him to give me a ring?"

Stella nodded wordlessly. The smoke cloud above her head spiralled around, slowly and steadily.

Frank sat with hands wrapped around a steaming cup of coffee. It was weak — barely drinkable — but kept the icy air whipped up from the River Mersey from numbing his fingers. He squinted his eyes as the wind started to burn his rosy cheeks and a weather-induced tear ran down the side of his face. The iconic Mersey ferry stuttered across the choppy waters, packed with commuters and visitors seeking a unique perspective of the famous skyline.

Frank felt the metal bench vibrate, but he didn't need to turn his head.

"I thought you'd be here," said Stan, who'd taken a seat beside him. "Not sure about this coffee," he remarked.

Frank didn't speak, but smiled.

"We were worried about you, Frank. Stella has been all over the place when you didn't turn up."

Frank's smile opened up into a gentle laugh. "Now I know you're lying," he said.

"Not about the coffee, though," said Stan, emptying the contents into a salty puddle near his foot.

The two of them sat in silence as the minutes passed by like the ships heading out into the Irish Sea. It wasn't uncomfortable, but without saying anything, it was poignant, almost comforting. Frank used his hand to push his hair down which was being tossed about in the breeze. He wiped another tear teased out from the wind off his cheek and turned to look at Stan.

"You've had your hair done?" he asked. Stan's hair was full of 'product' and in spite of the gale force wind, and unlike Frank's struggle to keep his own sorted, not a strand was out of place.

Stan nodded at the question. "Yes," he replied. "Although I'm starting to regret it. Stella's been taking the piss, and to be honest, I look like a bloody Oompa Loompa with this tan. What did the doctor say?"

"He said you look like an Oompa Loompa as well," Frank managed.

Of course, he knew what Stan was asking. Frank hadn't thought about his appointment since Stan had arrived, actually, and the question startled him. It brought him back to reality and his shoulders dropped. He looked at Stan and with a feigned smile he slowly shook his head. The sporadic tears were now replaced with a constant stream and his shoulders began to convulse.

"Oh, shit, pal."

Stan placed one hand on Frank's knee before moving closer, putting his arms around his shoulder.

"Everything I want to say to you right now is a cliché, and I mean everything. Frank, you know I'm here for you, no matter what. You know that, don't you?"

Frank tapped Stan's knee in acknowledgement.

"I know, Stan. We've been through quite a lot these last few years. Still... it's not been all bad today. I found her in bed with Boris, and I told her it's over."

"Poor bloke," said Stan.

Frank smiled. "You mean, Boris, don't you?"

"Absolutely, the guy deserves a medal," replied Stan. "And you can stay with me, I insist."

"I'm glad you said that because I've already been round to yours and left a couple of bags in your garage."

"A bit presumptuous!" said Stan.

"I knew you wouldn't see me on the street. Come on, let's walk a while," said Frank, shaking his arms to get the blood flowing back to his fingers. He turned for a moment and looked up to the peak of the Royal Liver Building towering above them.

Stan buttoned up his coat as they walked directly into the roiling wind. The two of them stopped and looked down on an empty berth, and a sign posted for the Isle of Man Ferry. "I used to love coming down here as kids, packed up and ready for our summer holidays," he said. "It's funny, as I look back on it, through a child's eyes, it never rained, the sea was never rough, and you just seem to filter out the negativity. Do you remember our mums would give us a few coins to get sweets for the crossing over, and most of the time we'd have eaten them by the time we got onto the boat?"

"I remember getting a clip across the ear when I'd be tapping my sister up for a few of her sweets," laughed Frank. "It's strange, but when I come down here and the ferry isn't in, I feel a bit... sad. I don't know why, perhaps it's the disappointment that we're not six again, all going on our holiday. How many times did we go to the Isle of Man?"

Stan thought for a moment.

"I'm not sure, it must have been eight or nine years on the trot. I remember feeling guilty, complaining to my parents that I didn't want to go in the end. I'd give everything I own to be stood here right now, you with your family and me with mine, bags in hand and ready to spend our two weeks on the Isle of Man... and now it's only me and you that's left."

"Bloody hell, Stan. Are you not meant to be cheering me up? I feel like jumping the Mersey now."

Frank thought a moment before continuing.

"I wish I'd taken my family over there, but they weren't interested. If there wasn't a cocktail bar and white sand, she was never interested. It's a shame, because our Molly has missed out on the things we used to do. Still, I suppose it was a different time and kids of her generation probably wouldn't have enjoyed that sort of holiday. Or, maybe that's why I get sad looking at the docks — because I didn't take her on that sort of holiday. It was all long-haul, but that was to please her mother...

"Maybe I should have been more insistent, and then perhaps she wouldn't have turned out quite as materialistic as she is. You know what Stan, you and I had nothing. Our parents probably saved up all year to take us on that boat and get us in that boarding house, and there was always money for an ice cream or a bag of chips when we got there. I can still picture your mum and mine sat on the promenade eating candy floss and our dads coming from behind and pushing it into their faces...

"It was simple pleasures back then. I miss that, Stan, I really do."

Stan looked at Frank with purpose. "Let's do it," he said.

"What?"

"The Isle of Man, let's do it. For old time's sake," said Stan, getting more animated.

Frank curled his nose up for a moment, but the frown turned steadily to a grin.

"Come on!" insisted Stan. "Look, don't take this the wrong way, but you're now technically eligible for a bucket list, are you not? And this could be the first trip on our bucket list."

"Our bucket list?" asked Frank.

Stan looked offended. "Damn right, our bucket list, you selfish old bugger. I'm not letting you do it on your own. If I had a terminal illness, I'd bloody well let you come on my list. I'm coming, and that's that."

Frank's face lit up. "We could afford to travel anywhere in the world, first-class, and you want us to go to the Isle of Man?" he asked.

"What fun is first-class? And besides, I know you too well, you're not first-class material, you're as common as muck. We can get the boat over, stay at a small B&B, and revisit the places we went as kids. You always wanted to see the TT Races. We could do that. And we *should* do that!"

"What about work?" asked Frank.

"Who are you kidding? Stella doesn't even know we're there most days, she'll hold the fort for us." Stan took his mobile phone and searched for the TT schedule. "Right. Here we go... last week in May and the first week in June. We can go for practice and race week. This is getting booked!"

Frank put his hand on Stan's shoulder. "Thanks, Stan," he said. "I mean it. There's no one I'd rather spend time with on my bucket list than you. Though I'm only coming to the Isle of Man if you give me a couple of quid to buy some sweets for the journey over."

"Done. But only if you promise not to eat them before the boat leaves! Come on, let's go and get you settled in. It'll be weird, me and you living together — we'll be like the *Odd Couple*."

"Stan," Frank interjected, looking concerned. "I'm not sure the sea air agrees with your fake tan... it looks like your face is melting."

"Don't take the piss," said Stan. "If you're staying with me then you're getting a fake tan as well."

"Do I need to get enough tacky gold to make Mr T jealous, also?" asked Frank.

"Cheeky bugger. Just because you're dying, doesn't mean I won't kick your arse," said Stan as they walked away from the pier head. "Me and you on the high seas, going to the TT races... I cannot bloody wait. See if you die before we go, I'll bloody kill you!"

chapter three

a fly crawled up the inside of the glass chiller cabinet, in no hurry at all, seemingly so full that it made no attempt to feast on the platter of tired-looking salad assortments below. It couldn't even be bothered to land and vomit, apparently, so languid was it in its sated state.

Its progress had not gone unnoticed by Eric Fryer, proprietor of the skilfully-thought-out Fryers Café. He moved gracefully — like a cheetah stalking a gazelle — and in a flash, he took the off-white dishcloth draped over his shoulder and unleashed it like a whip. The sound of the contact of fabric hitting surface was properly satisfying, and the proprietor bowed his head inside the cabinet as if saying a prayer for the deceased.

"Good shot, Eric, you got it," said Frank, who'd been looking on in mild amusement.

"It didn't fly away?" asked Eric, head still lowered. He wasn't praying after all. "I can't seem to find the little fucker."

"No," said Frank, sat at one of the four tables closest to the cabinet. "You got it, I can see the remnants of the wing and the contents of its stomach are now etched on the inside of your cabinet."

"Ah. I'd been looking low when I should've been looking high."

Rather than reach for a cloth to remove the fly-related detritus, Eric walked around to the front to admire his precision. "Indiana Jones would have been proud of that one, waddaya reckon?" he announced. "Did Hannah take your order, Frank?"

Frank shook his head, "No, not yet, Eric. I think I'll probably give the salad a miss, though."

"Yeah, I would too," said Eric, who'd now seen that the fly's other wing had landed on top of a tub of coleslaw that had the first appearances of a crust forming on it. "What can I get you, Frank?" he asked cheerfully.

"Just toast and a cup of tea. Thanks."

Frank looked at his watch and then to his phone.

"Stan not with you today?" asked Eric.

"No, I'm meeting my daughter. Well. Supposed to be, at any rate," said Frank, looking at his watch once again. "Punctuality was never one of her most endearing features."

Hannah took to making Frank's order, leaving Eric to hover, looking uneasy.

"How's, eh... how's Stella?"

Frank looked confused. "Fine, I think. But she's not exactly an open book. Why do you ask?"

"Nothing," Eric replied instantly. "Just wondered."

Frank screwed up his face. "You haven't... you and Stella?"

"What, no, of course not," Eric said, looking over his shoulder to ensure Hannah was out of earshot, and then pulled up a chair opposite and moved his head closer. "Well, yes, but don't let Hannah know, she can't stand Stella, and she'll just take the piss."

"You... and Stella?" said Frank, with a similar reaction to seeing the fly implode. "I'm not sure who I feel sorrier for. How long's that been going on for?"

"Not long, Frank. She comes in here every morning for her fry-up, with extra bacon. I caught her giving me the eye and I asked her out."

"You sure she was giving you the eye and it wasn't just wandering? Because her right eye is lazy and doesn't point in the same direction as the other. Or is it her left eye?" said Frank, raising his head to picture her face.

"I've always liked them with a bit of meat on the bones," explained Eric. "Gives you something to get a grip off."

"Thanks, Eric, I think I get the picture."

"So, she didn't mention me?" pushed Eric.

"No... can't say she did, Eric, but I'll be sure to put a good word in if she asks about you."

Eric stared into space with a simple grin on his face, "Great... great, thanks, Frank, what a wonderful night," he said, evidently recalling an evening of romance. "She's a special girl, Stella."

Frank was eager to end the conversation, but sometimes you just have to go with it. "So... you took her out for a meal, or something?"

"No, we went to the cinema. Well, it'd already started so they wouldn't let us in. I said I'd take her to Nando's but she said she'd be happy with a Mars Bar and can of Lilt fizzy pop. She took me round the back of Tesco's — on the high street — and gave me the best hand-job I've ever had."

Frank grimaced and thought he might well be ill. "How's that toast coming on, Hannah? Hannah!" he said desperately.

Two burly-looking builders opened the door just then, and it was back to business, thank goodness. And give Eric his due, he knew exactly what they wanted before they'd opened their mouths. He knew appetites.

Frank could see Molly crossing the road and moved to take the table closest to the window. She caught a glimpse of him and scowled in his direction.

Molly barged through the door — almost taking it off the hinges — and looked around the small café with contempt.

For a spring day, it was relatively mild, but the microscopic skirt and painted-on shirt were not really in keeping with the season, with most still sporting a heavy coat. The two builders were quick to make their appreciation known, smiling as Molly took a seat. Good money had been paid for that chest they were admiring, and she was apparently determined to get maximum exposure from it.

She threw her bag on the table.

"What are you doing, are you having some sort of delayed, mid-life crisis?" she said shortly.

"You're doing that thing that really annoys me, Molly," replied Frank. "You know. When you're shouting at me, but you do it as if you're actually talking, but it looks like and sounds like you're actually shouting? *That* thing. It's really annoying."

"What are you doing bringing me to this... this *dump*," she said, looking around once again. "My clothes are going to smell like fried egg."

She caught one of the builders staring over at her, and flicked her shoulder-length hair whilst flashing him the faintest of smiles.

"And what the hell is this nonsense that you've walked out on Mother?"

"Mother? Since when did you start calling her *Mother?* And stop shouting at me like I'm a child, please. I tried to tell you yesterday, but you didn't pick up your phone. I'm sorry you didn't hear it from me first."

Molly's amateur dramatics were increasing. She was twenty, but exceptionally immature, even if she didn't think so herself.

"My god, Dad, this is so embarrassing. If my friends find out you've walked out on Mother, I'll be a laughingstock. It's bad enough that they think you're..." she said, her voice trailing off.

"Yes? That I'm *what*, exactly?" Frank said. "That I'm a taxi driver, Molly?"

Molly didn't respond, but did briefly take a more conciliatory tone as the tea and toast were delivered to the table. She gave Hannah, the waitress, a condescending smile.

"Do you want something to eat?" asked Hannah.

Molly barely hid her look of disgust at the suggestion, but then relented.

"Dad, any recommendations?"

"The salad," replied Frank instantly. "Definitely the salad."

"The salad it is," said Molly.

"With chips?" asked Hannah. "Or, I could put a fried egg on the side...?"

"Mmm, I think I'll just stick with the salad, but, thanks for asking," said Molly, in her condescending tone which came so easy it was almost natural.

Frank cleared his throat. "I need to talk to you about something, Molly. It's important."

She wasn't listening. She'd removed a diamanté-encrusted compact mirror from her bag and admired her perfectly-applied makeup. She was also using the reflection to covertly look at the younger of the two builders to make sure he was still staring in her direction. He was.

Like the flick of a switch, and ignoring her father's announcement, her tirade continued.

"I don't understand you, Dad. Mother is stunning, and, this may come across as mean, but for someone your age, having a woman looking like that, well, are you stupid or something? Most men would kill for a wife like that."

"Most men would kill *if* they had a wife like that," Frank mumbled under his breath, though not loud enough so that his daughter could hear. He was resisting the overwhelming urge to tell her what her mother was really like. He'd run through this meeting in his head, several times, and was determined to retain an air of dignity.

"Are you cheating on her?" asked Molly.

Frank screwed up his face. "Good god, no, of course I'm not," he said. "Why would you even think that?"

Molly was barely listening once again. She had a habit of asking a question without being overly interested in the response. Her attention was now taken by turning her nose up at the décor in the café. She had her arms rested on the table, picking at its ageing, flaking varnish like a scab.

Hannah placed the most pathetic-looking salad imaginable onto the table. "Is there anything else I can do for you, or do you have everything you need?" she asked Molly. Getting no response, she shrugged and walked away.

"I just don't understand this," Molly said, finally.

"What, the salad?" Frank asked.

"You've got a beautiful home," she continued, her train of thought passing straight past her father's joke without slowing or stopping. "Money in the bank. Why would you walk out and leave her like this? How could you do it to her? You're just selfish, Dad."

"I'm bloody selfish, is it?" Frank said, the flag dropping and his anger charging. "You've got to be joking. Do you know what it's been like for me living with your mother? Do you have any idea? The only thing she's cared about is what people think of her — or, more importantly, what people think of *me* — if we're doing well enough, and properly keeping up appearances."

"She loves you, and wanting the nicer things in life is not a good reason to walk out on her. You're tearing this family apart."

"Bloody hell, Molly!" said Frank loudly. "Look, I didn't want to tell you this, but I caught your mother in bed with her fitness instructor!"

Molly did not respond to this, not as one should expect.

"You can work on your marriage," she insisted. "You can both recover from this."

Frank screwed up his face again. "Your mother threw a pair of leather underpants at me, with a strap-on dildo attached," he said. "A *vibrating* strap-on dildo. That sort of thing you do not recover from," he said animatedly, his voice juddering.

"Boris is just a phase," Molly said flippantly. "Surely you've cheated on *her*..."

"No. No, not once have I cheated on your mother. I wouldn't do that."

Frank took a mouthful of his tea.

"Hang on, how do you know about Boris? And how do you know it's just a phase?"

Molly flicked the limp-looking lettuce with her tarnished fork. "Mum told me she had a fitness instructor. Called Boris."

"You're avoiding the question, Molly. Everyone knows she has a fitness instructor called Boris — she was very insistent on telling people — but you said it was a *phase*. So you must have known your mother was sleeping with him?"

Molly bowed her head like a guilty dog.

"Who else knew about them?" asked Frank, but then quickly changed his mind. "Oh, you know what, it doesn't matter. There are more important things to worry about than them two, and to be honest, I'm beyond caring. They're welcome to each other."

"Dad, I'm worried about you. If you leave her in the house, where are you going to live? You should go back to her."

Frank smiled. "I know exactly what you're worried about. You're panicking that I'm going to chuck you out of the penthouse apartment you've been living in rent-free for the last twelve months. Don't worry, Molly, I wouldn't dream of being so selfish...

"Look, Molly, there is something I need to tell you, but I want to do it in a calm manner. I don't want you to think I'm doing it while I'm angry to score points—"

Molly raised one finger to silence him as she reached for her phone.

"Hi, Sue," she said, listening for a moment.

She mouthed an apology to her father.

"Yes, I can be there in five minutes," she said into her mobile.

She put the phone to her chest and picked up her bag.

"Dad, I've got to go, sorry." She kissed him on top of the head. "You'll be fine, Dad. If I can do anything, just let me know."

She put the phone back to her ear and continued her conversation. "Hmm? Oh, he's fine," she said, walking out the open door. And then, after a short pause, "Oh, no... he said I can stay there. So, yay!"

Out on the pavement, she walked past the window where Frank was sat with a renewed spring in her step, giving him a half-wave as she left him there.

Eric had his elbows resting on the counter and waited until Frank caught his eye.

"Frank, I might be out of order saying this, but your daughter, she's a bit of..."

"Selfish cow?" said Frank.

"Well, yes. She didn't even eat her salad."

Frank smiled. "Probably a good thing, Eric. Otherwise, you'd be up on a manslaughter charge."

Frank took his mobile phone and held his thumb over the keypad. He chewed the inside of his cheek and screwed his eyes up, deep in thought. Eric brought him back by appearing beside him and freshening his cup. Frank smiled and placed a single sugar cube into the steaming drink. The cubes were probably only a little more expensive than a sachet, but somehow they always made the tea taste better. Frank struggled to hear as another stream of hungry workmen stomped into the café.

Frank stuck a finger in his ear as the phone rang. "Yes, hello, Harry? Harry, It's Frank..."

"... Yes, I've just been with her," he continued, "No, I've not changed my mind."

Frank fidgeted with the metal tongs in the sugar bowl as he listened for a moment, and then, "Harry, I want you to start the divorce proceedings."

He'd thought about saying that phrase countless times over the years, but now he'd said it, it brought no relief. Saying it aloud made it real, but it was tinged with a sense of defeat — a feeling that something he'd worked on for years was a failure.

"The doctor?" asked Frank. "The doctor. No, it wasn't the best news."

Frank took a mouthful of the tea, which burned his lips.

"Harry, I'm not ready to talk about it just yet, to be honest. I'm going to start the treatment, and see how I get on. I don't want to advertise the fact, and I know I don't need to tell you, but, there are only a couple of people that know, and I'd prefer to keep it that way."

Frank nodded his head until the furrows in his forehead intensified. "Thought about my will? Bloody hell, Harry, you know how to cheer someone up."

His face returned to normal, the furrows relaxing and a warm smile appearing.

"I know, Harry. I'm just pulling your leg. I know you're only looking out for me, as you've done for twenty years. I know I said I didn't want to make it difficult for her, but, I don't. I've no desire to spend the next few months fighting with her. We should give her an offer that will make her go away quietly...

"The house?" said Frank. He thought for a moment. "Give her the house, and change the will so that the apartment goes to my loving daughter."

Frank listened for a bit.

"Harry, I know what you're saying. I know she cheated on me and I could make it difficult, but she's the mother of my child, one who is going through a challenging phase, but still, she gave me a daughter. I can buy another house. I just want

33

her out of my life. Oh, Harry, one more thing, will you speak with the accountants? I want to cash in some of my investments...

"How much? I don't know," said Frank, chewing his cheek once again. "I'm just going to take some time off work and have a bit of fun. I'm going to work through my bucket list, and from what Stan's saying, he's joining me."

Frank started to laugh.

"No, I don't think we need sun cream and leopard-skin Speedos where we're going first. We're going to the Isle of Man. I don't think it gets that hot there."

chapter four

Stan used the well-thumbed copy of the paper — stolen from the waiting room — to waft away the smoke emanating from Stella. He sat back in his cream-leather reclining chair that was stained tobacco yellow, like Stella's index finger.

"Is Frank on the grid, yet?" shouted Stan. There was no immediate response, so he wheeled the chair to the small window and repeated his question. "Let me know when you see him!" he shouted.

"I've not seen the lazy bugger all week?" responded Stella in a gruff voice. "Anyway, I thought he was living with you since he binned off that plastic-looking tart."

"He is living with me, but he's been a bit mysterious. Ah. Don't worry, I've just seen his car pull up on the lane."

"Ask him if he's going to grace us with his presence and actually do some work!" commanded Stella.

Stan had considered telling her about Frank's current medical issues, but compassion had never been one of Stella's strongest points.

"Where have you been?" asked Stan, as Frank made his entrance. "And why are you wearing a tracksuit?" Frank was normally well turned out, so to see him in tacky-looking sportswear was unusual.

He had a grin on his face as he collapsed into his seat, opposite Stan.

"I've been to a nude life drawing class, and thoroughly enjoyed it," said Frank proudly.

"You don't draw?" said Stan.

Frank popped the plastic lid of a cardboard roll and removed a piece of A4-sized paper.

"I know I don't, but I know people who can. And draw very well, as it would appear."

He passed the sheet to Stan, who took his reading glasses from the table. He looked at the paper and then peered over the top at Frank.

"It's you, Frank."

"I know it is, Stan."

"But you're naked," said Stan, taking another look.

"I know I'm naked. You don't tend to wear clothes at a nude life drawing class."

Stan placed his fist up to his mouth and bit the meat between the thumb and forefinger. It was clear he was trying to make sense of this in his mind but was having difficulty.

"She's certainly caught my good side," Frank carried on cheerfully. "Although I think she's overexaggerated the size of my stomach."

Stan cleared his throat. "I'm not sure that's the only thing she's been overly generous with."

Frank grinned. "I know, it's impressive. I was worried the room might be a bit cold and I wouldn't do myself justice, but she must have been impressed with the merchandise because she asked me out for a drink."

"Placing that aside," said Stan. "Why are you stripping off in front of strange women?"

Frank took the picture from Stan's hands, which Stan looked only too willing to let go, and carefully rolled it back into its cardboard tube.

"It's your fault, actually," he said. "With this trip to the Isle of Man, you got me thinking about other things I hadn't done. Hadn't done, and wanted to."

Stan shrugged his shoulders. "Call me old-fashioned," he said. "But I think a bucket list is supposed to be things like swimming with dolphins, soaring above the Serengeti in a hot air balloon, or snake charming. Not getting your tackle out in front of strangers in an old church hall."

"Sometimes you need to set your sights a bit higher," said Frank.

"Yes, well, surely this is setting them rather lower?" asked Stan. "I mean—"

"I milked a cow yesterday," interrupted Frank.

"What? Why?"

"I've never done it, that's why, so I thought, *that's what I'm going to do*, so I did."

"Yes, but why would you want to—?"

"Now I can say I've milked a cow," said Frank, well chuffed.

"Did you enjoy it?" asked Stan.

"Udderly," replied Frank.

Stan groaned. "Tell me you didn't just..." Stan caught a glimpse of Stella, who pushing herself out of her chair.

"Look, Stella's coming in. I've not told her about your trip to the doctor, so she thinks you've been dodging work. You should hide that picture, because if she sees you naked, she'll want to charm your snake."

"Where have you been all week, you lazy shite?" Stella, now stood in the doorway, said without invitation, shouting over to Frank. The filter of her cigarette was stuck to her bottom lip so, when she spoke, it waggled lewdly from the movement of her lips.

Frank stared at her for a moment, "Stella, you've got a half-eaten doughnut stuck to your leg."

Stella had a habit of wearing leggings and clothes that were, being kind, not suited to a woman with a figure so... voluminous. She looked down, but had to arch her neck as her stomach obstructed her view. She brushed the sugar off her leggings and scratched a patch of crusty jam that had been securing the abandoned treat in place before repeating the question once again. You'd be entirely forgiven for thinking she was in charge, the way she chastised Frank for his absence.

"I'm sorry, Stella," Frank offered. "I have been a bit slack this week."

"It's not good when the drivers see you two taking the piss," Stella admonished. "It makes them think they can start to skive. I'm trying to keep them all in line, but when you're swanning about, doing god knows what, and it's not good for discipline."

"You're quite right, Stella. And Stan and I appreciate the work you do. Look, I wasn't going to say anything, but I think I should..." said Frank, looking over at Stan.

"I've been to the doctors, see?" he continued. "And it wasn't the greatest news, I'm afraid," he said, nodding his head toward his midriff.

Stella sucked the life out of the remnants of the cigarette as she scratched her chin. She stubbed out the cigarette into the remains of the doughnut, which was still in her hand. "Ah, I see," she said sympathetically. "No lead in the old pencil, is it? Softer than a wet biscuit? You wouldn't have that problem with me, yeah? I've never had a man struggle to get the flag up the pole — it's an art form," she said, plucking and tugging absently at a segment of her leggings that had retreated too far up into a dark crevasse of no return.

"Is that why she left you? Fed up of the limpness?"

Frank took a moment to collect himself.

"Firstly, Stella. I'm pleased that you're so accomplished at giving men an erection, but I can assure you that I've no problem in getting little Frank to attention when required."

"Show me," she said immediately.

"What? I'm not bloody showing you that."

"We're friends," continued Stella. "And if you need me to help you rise to the occasion, you just need to ask."

She pushed her elbows toward each other — which further enhanced her already prodigious cleavage — as she slowly gyrated like an Indian belly-dancer.

"Say the word, Frank and I'll have you harder than a woodpecker's lips."

Frank took a step back, and found, unfortunately, that he could retreat no further.

"That's, well... very kind, Stella. And reassuring. But that's not the problem, honestly. It's actually a bit more serious than that. The doctor gave me some news that wasn't the least bit good, and, well... it's caused me to take stock of my life...

"Oh, and another thing. I left *her*, she didn't leave me!"

Stella stared for a hard moment before walking toward Frank. She took his head firmly in her hands and thrust his head into her chest.

Frank felt himself falling, falling, and wondering when his head's pillowous descent would come to an end.

She held him for a lingering, tender moment.

Frank started to struggle for air.

She stroked the back of his head, and made reassuring noises like a mother caring for a child.

"We're family," she said. "If you need me for anything, you just ask, and if you're missing female company, just phone me and if I'm available I'll be straight over."

She was certainly an unusual and often misunderstood woman, but it was clear that her intentions were genuine.

"I'll be sure to call, Stella," said Frank, struggling to catch his breath as he was finally allowed to come up for air.

"Anything!" she repeated once more, extending her thumb and pinkie finger from her chubby fist, making the shape of a phone, and waggling it against the side of her face, thumb against her ear.

"Now there's an offer for you," said Stan as soon as she was comfortably out of earshot and left the room. "Have you told your family yet?"

"About Stella's offer? Don't be daft. And she's only just made it besides. And you don't seriously think..."

But then Frank understood what Stan was really on about.

"... Oh. I have. Well. I've told Molly — was finally able to tell her — so no doubt her mother will now know as well. She cried, Molly, which surprised me."

"Well, she is your daughter, Frank."

"I know, but it's been a long time since she was my little girl, but when she was upset, for a fleeting moment, it was like she was my little girl again. Her mother will no doubt be rubbing her hands at the prospect of me shuffling off my mortal coil, or perhaps I'm doing her a disservice?"

Stan slapped the newspaper he'd been holding onto down on the desk. "Is that why you're intent on giving your cash away? Stop her from getting her grubby fingers all over it?"

Frank was confused until he caught sight of the front page:

Mystery Benefactor Pays to Feed City's Homeless

Frank tried to continue with the confused expression. He had felt a bit like Bruce Wayne from Batman, but his alter ego had been uncovered at the first hurdle.

"How did you know that was me?" he asked.

Stan smiled. "I didn't. It was a guess, but sounded like something you'd do in your current state of mind."

Frank scoured the paper, making sure his name wasn't mentioned. "It wasn't that expensive, it was food vouchers for a couple of hundred people," he said. "I've paid for the next three years. Keep it between me and you, please. Yeah?"

"Of course. And that's good of you," said Stan. "And I cannot wait to hear Helen's reaction when she knows her divorce settlement is feeding the homeless!"

Frank gave a wry smile. "I'll try and capture the moment on my phone. Just for you, anyway," he said, looking at his watch.

"Somewhere to be?" asked Stan.

Frank nodded. "I've booked a Jet Ski lesson. On the Mersey. Something I've always wanted to do."

"That'll be bloody freezing!" said Stan. "Still, a bit more aspirational than milking a cow. If you like that sort of thing, I suppose," he continued. "And it's your arse on the line, not mine, after all, thank goodness for that."

Stan chuckled to himself as he picked the newspaper up from Frank's desk and tucked it up under his arm for a read later on. "I'll save this for my late-afternoon bowel movement," he said. "Frank, you ever notice *bowel movement* sounds like a symphony?" he continued dreamily. "Bowel Movement in A Minor. What do you reckon? Heavy on the horn section, I expect."

Frank walked towards the door, but then turned round. "Right, I wouldn't get too comfy if I was you, Stanley, me old mate," Frank said, breaking Stan's reverie. "That lesson I've booked is for the two of us, mind you. After all, you're the one who said he wanted to share my bucket list. So, you're sharing this!"

"What? I'm not going into the bloody Mersey River!" replied Stan, laughing nervously. "I'm not a keen swimmer, you know, and it'll be brass monkeys!"

"You swim like a dolphin."

"They kill dolphins in Japan, you know! I've seen it in a documentary!" Stan protested.

"You're just worried that the sea will wash off your fake tan," said Frank. "Come on, get your coat, we're going jet skiing and that's the end of it."

There was nothing more to be said. Stan grabbed his coat as instructed.

"Dolphins can sleep with half their brain at a time, did you know that?" Stan added as they walked out the door. "So they're always alert. They're very clever animals."

And then they were off.

chapter five

Liverpool City Centre was, as usual, a hive of activity. It was just after midday and a continuous stream of tourists, shoppers, and workers — on their lunch hour — filled the streets like industrious ants. It wasn't difficult to be anonymous in this sprawling metropolis. For many, the ability to blend in and be just another face was appealing. But there were those who longed to spot a friend in the crowd and have a welcoming, compassionate glance thrown their way.

Lee Watson was one of those lost souls.

He sat in an uninspiring doorway that was cloaked with the rancid smell of stale urine but could equally be radiating from his own clothing. His head was bowed at waist height to those passing by and he held a discarded McDonald's milkshake cup loosely in his hands, shaking it periodically. He'd become accustomed to the looks of contempt thrown in his direction over the months, and found it easier to stare vacantly at the ground below him. The ruthless cold of the winter had fortunately passed and the longer, warmer days were beginning to return.

He didn't have friends, but rather acquaintances who were in a similar position to his, with some moving on, perhaps some enjoying a change of fortune or reunited with family. But some, particularly the older ones, had succumbed over the colder months. While he didn't drink to excess, he could understand those that did; for some, it was the only way to escape the harsh reality of their existence — at least for a short while.

"Spare change, sir," he said half-heartedly, to no one in particular.

Lee had long since given up expecting a response, or money placed in his cup, and once again he wasn't disappointed.

He wasn't stupid. He was personable, and he'd worked for years, so the hardest point to digest about his current situation... was how the hell he'd ended up in this current situation. He had no money in his pocket and no idea where his next meal was coming from. His only possessions were the clothes he wore and a blanket and pillow which he carried in a backpack.

Of course, he wanted more than this. But the more you had, the more likely you'd be robbed of those possessions. If you accumulated anything, you had to be prepared to fight to retain them, and he was fed up of fighting. He'd seen people prepared to take a life over a bottle of cider or a premium place to sleep out of the cold. There were those that had resigned themselves to this life. But, for most, they were desperate to escape from the sheer hopelessness. Lee was desperate and was struggling to drown out the droning in his head telling him to jump from a tall building. If he had to face the prospect of another winter, especially, he felt he'd most certainly give in to the incessant voice buzzing around in his skull.

He looked up briefly to survey the volume of passing people; if quiet, he'd move on to another bolthole. A small boy, three, maybe four years of age, stared intently at Lee as his mother pulled tightly on his hand. The boy didn't look away, even as he passed, and struggled further with his mother before finally managing to break free of her grasp.

The boy walked up to Lee, presenting him a lolly, in his hand, that he clearly treasured but was nevertheless willing to part with.

"I've only licked it twice," the child assured him. "It's still good."

Lee smiled warmly. That one small gesture had just made up for months of degradation.

The boy grinned back, until his mother came to retrieve him, yanking his arm and pulling him away from Lee.

"Don't speak to filthy losers like that!" she shouted in anger as they blended back into the crowd. Before he disappeared from sight, however, the little boy turned and smiled in Lee's direction once more, until, in the end, he was gone.

Those moments of kindness Lee had just experienced would now be tinged with the thought of being 'a filthy loser'.

He'd had enough. It wasn't that one incident that caused him to snap; rather, an accumulation, the pinnacle of a man who could take no more.

His cup had two coins in it and those were the ones he'd placed in it himself several hours earlier — to prime the pump, so to speak. He put the coins back in his pocket, put the lollipop in his mouth, and threw the cup on the ground.

He'd seen the security van every day, at the same time, for weeks. He thought it stupid that it came at the same time, almost to the minute. The guard was collecting the cash from some of the shops on the high street, and Lee had spent hours fantasising about grabbing that cash.

He was halfway across the street before he realised it. He had tunnel vision now — completely unaware what he was doing presently — the words *filthy loser* ringing in his ears, louder and louder.

His pace quickened and he'd given up avoiding the busy shoppers and now barged his way through them.

The security guard was returning to his van, carrying a large metal case, and cautiously looking at those in his vicinity as he'd no doubt been trained to do.

Call it instinct, but the guard caught sight of Lee marching toward him. But as he tried to react to the impending threat, Lee had now broken into a sprint.

The guard recoiled for a moment and tried to alert his colleague in the van, it seemed, but in an instant Lee had hurled himself through the air and dispatched both himself and the guard to the ground.

The shoppers nearby froze for a moment as they assessed the situation. Then they began to scream as the reality of it set in.

Those screams snapped Lee back to awareness, and he tried to right himself from the cold concrete floor. He looked up and could see fear in the guard's face.

But no sooner than he could blink than a second man appeared from nowhere, swinging a cricket bat. It just missed Lee, and, not the kind to take this sort of thing lying down, Lee grabbed for the man's leg, knocking him off balance. The man's botched attempt at robbery was scuppered further as the guard's companion, now at hand, was well prepared for a second volley with the wooden bat.

Lee was now focused on retreat and, for self-protection as well as good measure, kicked the bat-wielding man firmly in the bollocks, causing him to roar in agony and drop the weapon, which Lee immediately grabbed.

Lee struggled to his feet and ran, leaving the crease.

He had no idea where he was going, and just moved as fast as his feet would carry him. As soon as he'd moved away from the main shopping area, he threw the bat in the first available bin.

"Shit, shit, shit!" he said, struggling to regain his breath. "Bloody fucking hell!"

He continued walking as the sound of police sirens filled the air. He was stood in a small bay where the bins from a large supermarket were stored. As the sound of the sirens came closer, he jumped behind the nearest bin and cowered.

He stayed there for what felt like hours. He was consumed by the overwhelming feeling of guilt. He could never have lived with himself if he'd hurt that guard.

Lee had to eventually give in to the crippling pains of hunger and venture out from his pungent sanctuary. The cover of darkness put him at ease, but every time a police car passed, his heart smashed against his chest. He had no money to speak of and was desperate for food. He wanted to stay away from public areas, but the lure of a hot meal at the charity food bank was too strong.

Lee joined the small queue. He always admired the work of the volunteers who merrily dispensed meals to the desperate, with little reward other than a feeling of satisfaction, and he gratefully took a bowl of hot soup and a large sandwich. He sat in the corner of the room — ironically, a former police station that had been gifted to the charity — and tried to remain as inconspicuous as he could.

With the stinging hunger pains temporarily relieved, he dwelled with disgust on his earlier actions. He held his head in his hands as he thought about where to bed down for the evening. Through a gap in his fingers, he could see Tommy — the charity coordinator — scanning the collection the hungry patrons.

Lee sunk into his chair as low as was possible to sink as Tommy walked toward him, followed by two uniformed policemen. Lee considered making a run for it, but the idea of a room in a warm custody unit was now somehow very appealing.

"That's him," said Tommy, pointing in Lee's direction.

"Lee Watson?" asked the first officer, now before him. "Would you mind coming with us?"

Lee nodded.

"You can bring your sandwich if you like," continued the officer.

Lee was confused as to why he wasn't being wrestled to the ground and placed in handcuffs.

"Are you not arresting me?"

The policemen looked at each other in confusion.

"What? No, of course we're not. If anything, we should be buying you a pint!"

At which point they started laughing.

Lee laughed as well.

He had no idea why he was laughing, and it was the only thing that was stopping him from recycling his recent meal into his already filthy underpants. He thought he must have found himself in some sort of reality TV programme, and half expected a camera crew to jump out at any moment.

But no one jumped out at all.

It'd been months since he'd been in a car, and he — even in these circumstances — felt for a moment, more human. Even though Lee stank badly, the policemen politely said nothing. They merely wound their windows down slightly and moved their heads toward the fresh air.

"We'll get you a change of clothes at the station, maybe have a nice shower, Lee?"

Lee cleared his throat. "Erm, yes, thanks, that would be lovely."

He had no idea what was happening. He wondered for a moment if he'd knocked himself unconscious and was currently in a state of delirium.

At the police station, a brute of sergeant sat behind the custody desk. One of the officers who escorted Lee had a word in the sergeant's ear, and the sergeant's face changed from one dispensing justice to a warm, welcoming smile.

"Lee Watson, a pleasure to meet you. You'll get a civic award for your bravery. We've got the man in custody and just need to take a statement from you, if that's okay?"

"Sure," said Lee nervously, and still in the dark. They were either the most inept police force in the country, or knew something that he didn't.

Lee went with the second option. Lee took a step forward to the imposing desk. "You, erm... know what happened today, then?" he asked, gingerly.

The sergeant smiled. "CCTV, son. We've got the whole lot on video, which is why we knew who to look for. One of the guys recognised you as a street sleeper, so thought you may turn up at the shelter."

"Great!" said Lee. "Any chance I could... see it?"

"You want to see it?" the sergeant said, repeating Lee's words in a tone that was difficult to discern. It might have been suspicion, or it might have been nothing at all.

"I've, em, never seen myself on telly," Lee offered weakly, hoping the absurd excuse might somehow pass muster.

The sergeant shrugged his shoulders. "Don't see why not," he said amiably. "Gary, will you take him into the office and show him the footage?"

Lee sat uncomfortably as the CCTV footage appeared on the computer screen in front of him. The camera angle covered most of the street, and he smiled as the opening scene had captured the small boy handing him his lollypop.

He shifted uncomfortably in his seat, however, as the coverage showed him moving at pace toward the security guard. It was like watching a different person entirely. As he viewed himself approaching the guard, he could see a car appear at the corner of the screen and one man jump out of it. The images were a little grainy, but Lee could clearly see the man remove a cricket bat from the passenger seat of the car, walk past the security van, and march towards the security guard. Lee looked on while the man arched the bat behind his back and swung directly at the security guard... with contact only avoided by the actions of Lee, forcing the guard to the cement.

The coverage continued to show Lee wrestling with the man, before delivering a pinpoint accurate assault on the man's crotch — resulting in the man collapsing in a heap, right on the spot, like a building fallen under demolition once the explosive charges have gone off. Lee then observes himself on the screen as he removes the offending weapon from the assailant's possession, before finally retreating off-camera.

Watching the video back, Lee looked very much like bloody Batman keeping the streets of Gotham free from crime, with every move perfectly choreographed and strategically performed.

He looked like a hero.

And that's when he noticed the crowd of assembled police, who also been watching the video along with him, apparently, because when it came to end, they all cheered.

"Well done, mate!" shouted one of the officers.

"Guy's a hero!" shouted another.

Lee's shoulders were currently higher than they'd been for quite some while. He had the feeling that he may wake up at any moment, but he went with it.

He turned to the room and shrugged his shoulders. "Least I could do," he said with a grin, soaking up the admiration. Deserved or no, he'd take it. "I'm hardly a hero, though. Only I did what came naturally. Surely it's what anyone would've done?"

Lee saw his way clear to receive many claps on the back then, without complaint. It was the least he could do.

chapter six

"Sixty-two years young, Frank," said Stan, topping up his champagne flute. "Here's to many more!"

Frank smiled and took a grateful mouthful of the expensively inflated drink. "Thanks, but not sure there will be too many more, especially with my blood pressure in this place."

Stan scoured the room. "Yeah, it's not the place I quite remember. I don't think they've updated the furniture since I was last here years ago."

"I don't know about the furniture, but they certainly haven't updated most of the girls, honestly. Stella could get a job in here, looking at this lot."

Stan nodded.

"I'm not sure about a strip club, Stan," Frank continued. "It's not really my thing. Not anymore, at least. Probably something to do with having a wife and daughter spending my cash on fake knockers."

"Yeah, sorry, mate," Stan agreed. "It's a bit of a cliché to take out your newly single mate to a strip club. Should we just go the Lion for a couple of pints?"

Frank laughed as he looked around the strip club that was barely illuminated and tapped his foot along to the deliberately seductive music. He ran his hands on the fabric of the seat which was smooth, like cheap leather, and the realisation that the upholstery was designed to easily be 'wiped clean' encouraged him to finish his drink with increased gusto. He reached for his hat which sat — like a sleeping cat — on the shelf behind him.

The motion of his flailing hand was misinterpreted by a scantily-clad brunette as an invitation, or possibly request. She'd been circling the club like a hungry vulture and at the first indication of an easy meal, she flicked her hair seductively and arched her back to emphasise her already considerable attributes. She sauntered over, eyes locked on Frank.

Now presented before him, she gyrated slowly in time with the music, and for a lady with a fuller figure, one could say that she was certainly quite flexible.

Frank shifted uncomfortably, placing one hand down on the seat between his legs for leverage as he did so. The woman smiled at this, seeming to misinterpret Frank's discomfort as arousal.

"You like vhat you see."

She said this more as a statement than a question, and leaned over far enough so that her ample bosom, now on full display, brushed against the tabletop — never letting go of Frank's eyes as she did so.

Frank recoiled in his seat, much to the amusement of Stan.

"No," said Frank, not wishing to encourage her. "I mean, I'm sure you're lovely, perfectly lovely. But I wasn't asking for a dance, I was just reaching for my hat."

Her face turned to one of instant anger. *"You are for calling me fat?"* she shouted, over the din of the music.

Frank stuttered, "What? No. No, of course I didn't. No, no," he protested. "I said I was just reaching for my hat. *My hat.*"

She was placated and suggestively took the hat. "Ah. You are the cheeky boy," she said in broken English. "You vant me vear hat, da? Is no problem."

Frank was a little unsure what was happening as the woman — who'd introduced herself as Ivana — started to dance in front of him.

"Fifty pounds, lover," she said, drawing out the word 'lover' and pronouncing it as *loafer.* "You pay at end."

All Frank wanted was his hat back and a pint of bitter at the Lion, but at the risk of causing further offence, he went with it. She was now getting fully into her performance and her bra was now carefully placed on the seat beside him. She turned her back to Frank and playfully slid down his body, ending up on her knees. She turned once more to face Frank, and slithered back up his body until their noses were almost touching.

Ivana wasn't really having the intended effect, and Frank spent his time looking at the hat wondering if it was, in fact, really his style after all.

She held her proximity for a moment and Frank realised the thick application of perfume was also designed to mask the smell of alcohol, very likely gin. Fearing his hat was lost forever as a prop for her future performances, he made a concerted effort to retrieve it.

Unfortunately, Ivana took his sudden hand gesture as an attempt to bring their relationship to another level, and playfully slapped the back of his fingers.

"You very naughty!" she slurred.

Frank had heard before the song being played, and expectantly tapped his foot to the final bars of the music. Ivana surely knew, also, that these last notes were her cue to bring her performance to an end, and, apparently aiming to finish on a high, she crouched low — trying to grind her bum against Frank's crotch (a crotch which had remained blasé and unmoved throughout).

Her overindulgence, however, caused her to lose her balance and she fell back further than expected.

Ever the gentleman, Frank raised his hands, once more, to steady her fall, though the gesture was once again met with a dismissive slap on the wrist as the song came grinding, as it were, to a halt.

"Now you give Ivana fifty pounds," Ivana announced, eager, it would appear, to bring their transaction to a close and relieve Frank of the money he'd 'promised' her.

But there was a snag. As she tried to push herself into a standing position, she was prevented from doing so.

Frank assumed she'd drunk more than first assumed, and tried to help her back to her feet. Every time she made the effort to get to her feet, however, she immediately recoiled back to Frank's crotch like a spring.

At first, Frank thought it was perhaps an attempt to increase the payment due, until, with horror, he realised that the buckle on his belt had caught the lace on the back of her knickers. Every time she stood, the fabric stretched, catapulting her back to Frank's crotch.

After a half-dozen or so of these back-and-forths, the woman appeared, finally, to understand the physical nature of her dilemma. She turned her head and raised her voice in a language with which Frank found himself unfamiliar.

"No, stop," said Frank, who was now desperately pulling at his belt, but which only produced further chastising from Ivana.

"You need to stop pulling. Look!" he said, pointing furiously at his crotch, but his intentions were not received as they were intended.

The next swearword, Frank, along with the rest of the club, understood quite clearly, and she stood, this time, rather more forcefully.

The only option, Frank felt, to maintain the woman's limited modesty, was for him to stand also — whilst continuing the battle to release her from his belt.

They were now both stood, but as she was a touch shorter, Frank was now stooped over slightly. She moved frantically, as if trying to escape an angry wasp.

Everywhere she went, Frank went. She spun on the spot, and such was their coordinated movement that the uninitiated might be forgiven in thinking their dance had continued from the booth outside the allotted three minutes, and continued in a rather more enthusiastic, enflamed fashion.

There was a burly bouncer who, up to now, had stood politely, but firmly, policing those walking into the establishment. Frank and Ivana's wild gesticulations had caught the bouncer's attention, Frank noticed.

Ivana had noticed this as well, it seemed, as she presently moved toward the bouncer at pace, and, as a result, so did Frank — who continued to wrestle with her knickers.

The bouncer, now at hand, gripped Frank by the shirt and began to pry the two apart. "You've crossed the line, fella," he said.

Frank tried to protest and explain himself, grabbing hold desperately to Ivana's knickers, but it all happened too quickly, and Frank found himself fallen unceremoniously to the floor, still clutching the woman's knickers — separated from her body quite effectively in the process.

In the end, Ivana stood above him, her modesty now protected only by the bouncer's jacket.

"Pervert!" she shouted down at him.

Stan, who till this point had been an amused bystander, could feel the tension in the room and made an effort to interject.

"Look, it's his birthday!" was the best defence he was able to offer. "Lad's night out, yeah?"

Ivana looked indignant. "And, this means is OK to him for stealing knickers??"

"Well, you took his hat!" replied Stan, whose attention had suddenly moved elsewhere.

He was looking at a very attractive girl who emerged barely dressed from the darker recesses of the club. She moved closer and the look on Stan's face changed from shock to alarm.

"Dad! What the hell are you doing here? Are you mad? What are you playing at??"

The attractive young girl was now stood over him, hands on hips, looking down at him. She was topless, and had quite nice tits, though they didn't look entirely natural, Frank thought. Of course, they wouldn't. After all, he's the one who'd paid for them.

"It's not what it looks like, Molly!" protested Frank.

"Dad, you're lying on a strip club floor, with the buttons of your trousers wide open, holding a pair of knickers, next to a naked stripper. What the hell is it supposed to look like??"

Frank opened his mouth to answer, unsure of what he might say, but Molly wasn't finished.

"Oh, and I hope you got my card?"

Frank decided attack was the best form of defence.

"Never mind about me, what the hell are *you* doing here?"

Molly stamped her foot. "I'm bloody making a living, aren't I? You always told me to get a job, and so I've done. Besides, my boobs look fantastic, so why not?"

She pointed them in Stan's direction. "What do you reckon, Stan?"

"Em... very nice?" said Stan, uncertainly.

The bouncer appeared to have reached the end of his patience by this point, and visibly increased his body mass in frustration like an agitated pufferfish. "Right. You pair of tossers," he said. "Out of here, right now."

Neither Frank nor Stan needed asking twice, and Stan helped Frank up from the grubby carpet and they made for a hasty exit.

As they left, the bouncer held the door open to watch as they walked away, making sure, it would appear, that they'd well and truly gone.

"Shit!" said Frank. "I've forgotten my hat."

But Stan didn't stop to turn back.

"Alright, Indiana Jones, just leave it," Stan said. "You can buy another one with the fifty pounds you forgot to give to the stripper."

They moved swiftly away from the club, as Frank buttoned up his trousers. "I thought I was done for in there," he said.

Stan nodded, then took a look over his shoulder.

"Frank," Stan said wistfully. "Frank. Molly has got fantastic..."

"One more word, Stanley. Just one more word..." said Frank, who was still trying to take stock of the situation and convince himself that what had just happened had just happened.

The two friends walked through the City Centre and, throughout the walk, Frank was getting increasingly frustrated with the sporadic laughter coming from Stan. He knew he'd see the funny side of it all, eventually, but it wouldn't be tonight. Well, not until he'd had a couple of pints at the Lion, at least.

Living in a major city, Frank had always been aware of the homeless, but, like most, had become immune to their presence. Like once buying a new car, you only then become aware of how many of the same are on the road. And so, now, Frank was seeing homeless people everywhere.

He'd started to look at them differently. He wasn't seeing them as a pile of clothes in a doorway; these were real people with a story to tell. He wasn't stupid, he knew there were those that weren't good people and he knew the food voucher gesture of his could well fall into the hands of those undeserving, but he figured that, on the whole, he'd capture the good ones.

Frank took the £50 note in his pocket and walked toward a man sat in a shop doorway. The man didn't look hungry, or even particularly dirty. Rather, he looked lost. The expression on his face was one of hopelessness, like he'd given up. As Frank approached him, the man barely lifted his head.

Frank leaned down and handed the young man the note. "Take this and see what you can do with it," he said, barely stopping to see the reaction.

Stan looked puzzled upon Frank's return. "Was that a note you gave him?" he asked.

Frank nodded. "Yes, the money the stripper was going to get."

"Fifty bloody quid? You've more money than sense! Still, fair play to you," Stan said. "Look, Frank, this work with homeless..."

"What about it?"

"I'm in," said Stan. "I was really impressed with what you did with the food stamps, and, well, I'm in. I'd like to throw some money into the pot with you. Maybe help more people, for longer."

"The things you'll do when you're guilty for seeing my daughter's tits!" Frank laughed, and then, still smiling, put his arm around Stan. "Seriously, though, Stan. That's really good of you. I've had a few thoughts and I'd like to try and take it to the next level. Call it a legacy from a man facing the prospect of meeting his maker."

"Cheery thought," said Stan, but Frank had stopped behind him.

Stan turned around. "There you are," he said. "What are you doing?" he asked.

Frank was wracking his brain. "That man I've just given the money to. I'm sure I know him."

"You're a bloody taxi driver. You've probably met half of Liverpool," Stan offered.

"No, it's more than that," Frank said, and he paused for a moment longer before turning back to where they'd came.

Stan jogged to keep up. "What are you doing? Where are we going?" he asked.

The man in doorway saw Frank approach and stood.

"Look, mate, you've given me a fifty-pound note here. I was about to chase after you myself, in case it was your money to get home or something," he said, holding the note out to Frank.

Frank was touched at the gesture. The man spoke in a gentle, but strong Irish accent and judging by the less than svelte midriff, had clearly not been without a meal for too long.

"No, no, you keep it, please," said Frank, adding, "I don't mean to be rude, but did I not see you on TV last week?"

Stan moved closer. "It bloody is as well," he said. "You're the man that tackled the armed robber who had the baseball bat."

"Cricket bat," the man said. "And, well, I suppose I am," he added uncomfortably.

"Bloody hell, mate," said Stan, shaking his head sympathetically.

Frank nodded his head in agreement. "But, hang on, you did that last week and this week you're back to sleeping in doorways? I've got to be honest, when they said it was a homeless man who'd tackled the thief, I assumed he wasn't actually homeless and that the press had embellished the fact to make the story sound better."

"No, sadly, I am actually homeless," the young man said. "Well, at least at the moment. My name is Lee Watson, by the way."

"I'm Frank and this is Stan," said Frank, extending his hand. "Look, this might be a bit premature, but, well, I don't have a great deal of time."

"Bloody hell, Frank, stop being so negative," Stan said, annoyed.

"I don't mean that, Stan. It's getting near closing time, you tosspot, and I want a few pints!"

"Ah. Right, then," Stan said, chuckling.

"Lee, the thing is," Frank continued. "We're doing a bit of work with the homeless and want to try and extend what we can do. I'm not exactly sure what it will be, but, would you like a job?"

"Okay... that sounds good," Lee said hesitantly. "But... you don't know me. How do you know you can trust me?"

Frank smiled. "Well, you tried to give me my fifty pounds back without asking," he explained. "Now, as far as the job, I don't know where this is going to go, but it will give you a few quid in your pocket and get you back on your feet. Keep the money I already gave you, and take this as well," said Frank, handing him another £50. "Get yourself a room in the hotel over there, have a wash, and come and see me at this address tomorrow and we can talk further."

Frank wrote the office address down and handed it over.

Lee looked bewildered. "Thanks," he said. "But how will I get there?"

"Jump in any taxi with a picture of Frankenstein on the side," Frank said.

"Frankenstein's monster?" Lee asked, confused.

"Right. They'll bring you to the office," Frank explained.

Lee still looked confused.

"I'm Frank, see? And he's Stein," Frank said, pointing to Stan. "We just need to get him some bolts for the sides of his neck, is all."

Lee looked more confused.

"It's our taxi service," Frank said, explaining further. "We own the business."

Suddenly, a flash of realisation swept over Lee, animating his face. "Ah! Yes! I've seen them. With the monster on the side!"

"Frankenstein," said Frank proudly.

"Frankenstein's monster, yes," Lee said, nodding his head in agreement.

As Frank and Stan continued on their way, into the deserted shopping streets of Liverpool, a voice echoed off the brick walls along the lane, calling after them, booming like thunder from the reverberation.

"Thank you! Thank you both, very much! I won't let you down!"

Frank raised his arm in acknowledgement and placed the other around Stan's shoulder.

"We're going to do good things, Stanley. I'm looking forward to this!"

"Now let's go get that pint," Stan agreed.

chapter seven

the company ran an advert each year on regional TV. They were known for being low-budget, deliberately so, and often cringe-worthy bordering on self-deprecating. Frank had never been one for limelight. Stan, on the other hand, was a bon vivant who relished the opportunity to promote himself, and the lure of a leading role on small screen was one he was exceptionally eager to become involved with. His fake tan, dyed hair, and gregarious dress wouldn't have looked out of place in a 1970's American soap opera. On the adverts which had aired for years, Stan would appear with his usual flair, inevitably requiring rescue by one of their heroic taxi drivers in a ludicrously scripted situation where he needed a taxi. The strapline in the advert was: Frank 'n' Stan's – driven to help.

Stan had been grooming for days once Frank told him that BBC Breakfast were coming to do a live interview. His hair was now blacker than the Milk Tray Man on a moonless night, and he'd been a little too liberal with the application of his fake tan.

"It'll show up as a healthy bronzed glow on camera," he insisted.

The camera crew were due in just before 7 a.m. and the office was immaculate in anticipation. Stan had placed some sort of advert for the business at every conceivable angle and wore a t-shirt with their logo emblazoned all over it.

Every driver was given strict instructions that any impromptu appearances would be met with a severe beating, and Stella had never been out of her seat so much. For the third time that morning, she appeared with a cup of tea for Frank and Stan — despite having never made them a cuppa in the ten years prior, not once, not ever.

"Stella, you look different today," remarked Stan on her most recent trip.

Indeed, Stella's tight perm seemed more buoyant than usual and her leggings were almost indecent, like they'd been painted on. She certainly appeared proud of her new white t-shirt, which had the logo SWEAT IS JUST YOUR FAT CRYING stretched across the front. And though Stella never wore lipstick — likely because she had no lips to speak of, really — she wore it today, though without much in the way of lips, as noted, it had the appearance of a mouth having eaten its own lips, with her vibrant red lipstick, fag hanging through it, looking rather more like a traffic warning sign.

"Can a girl not make an effort?" she asked, dropping the two cups of tea onto the desk.

Frank caught sight of cigarette ash a moment before it sank beneath the surface of his drink, dissolving into the tea.

Stella stood for a moment and stared through the window, perhaps, one can only assume, looking for someone with a camera.

"I think that's the phone ringing," said Frank, with a smile on his face, and it wasn't just an excuse, either — the phone actually was ringing.

She didn't acknowledge him and continued to stare. "I've told my mum I'm going to be on the telly. So I don't want to let her down, understand?"

She looked at Frank and didn't blink. It was unnerving, and he looked toward Stan for help, but none was forthcoming.

"Well, Stella," he said. "The thing is, they're only really here to interview me and Lee. I hope you understand? It's to talk about the new charity, see."

She continued to stare.

"My mum will be watching," she said, breathing deeply and sucking in a lungful of toxic air.

Frank wafted the smoke away as best he could. "I'll see what I can do, Stella, but no promises. Also, if you don't mind, I'm not sure I need any help dying any quicker, so can you leave the smoking outside of the office, please?"

"That's a bit selfish," she said. "Especially as I've been making tea for you all morning."

She blew one final plume of smoke toward them and returned to the ringing phone.

Frank looked at Stan with a puzzled expression. "Why do we employ her, again?"

Stan pointed toward the sign above his head. *"If you need to phone in sick, remember you need to speak to Stella,"* it said.

"Because, Frank, as you know, without her, this place would be carnage."

Scarlett Redfern was captivating. She was the darling of BBC TV with a shock of auburn hair and a figure that would cause traffic to stop. As she marched with purpose into the taxi office, she brought an element of class never before seen in this particular environment.

"Frank?" she asked, as she approached, with a warm, engaging tone.

Frank and Stan were like two schoolboys. They weren't told who was coming to do the interview, and Frank mumbled an incoherent welcome. The camera crew were familiar with this reaction, and grinned as they set up their equipment.

Lee was late arriving, but forgiven, bearing in mind he was sleeping in an actual bed for the first time in months. Scarlett was a consummate professional, who put Lee and Frank at ease, positioning them for the most flattering light.

Stan would no doubt find himself delighted, as two of his strategically-placed adverts would remain in shot.

The cameraman, who was lining up the scene, raised his head, suddenly, from the view-finder.

"There's a woman in shot in the window," he said. Then he squinted his eyes. "I think it's a woman?"

Stella was staring through the window, and with the smoke surrounding her she looked like she'd just stepped out of the Tardis.

As Stella obviously had no intention of going anywhere, Stan very smartly closed the blinds.

Frank and Lee were wired up for sound as Scarlett touched up her immaculate makeup one final time before effortlessly going live to the camera.

Scarlett: I'm delighted to be with Frank Cryer and Lee Watson. Now, you may remember Lee, or will probably have seen him, as the homeless man who tackled an armed robber and now somewhat of an internet sensation. I'm very pleased to say that Lee is no longer homeless and is in fact working on a fantastic new charity venture. Frank, if I can come to you first? Can you let us know a little bit about the new venture?

Frank: Yes, thanks. It's something I only started fairly recently. This city has been good to me and the people have made our business thrive. I know a few people that have not had the best of luck in life, and sadly some of those have ended up on the streets. I wanted to do something to help them, so I put some money in so that the homeless can use their food stamps I've helped provide to go into a number of participating retailers to buy food.

Scarlett: Wow, that's a great initiative. So why now?

Frank: Ah, well, because I'm dying, and wanted to do something nice.

Scarlett went silent for a moment, expecting a punchline that was not forthcoming. The faces in the room were sombre, and for a moment she lost her composure before quickly righting herself.

Scarlett: I'm truly sorry to hear that, Frank. But this is a wonderful legacy. So, what's next?

Frank: My apologies, Scarlett, I didn't mean to throw that one in so matter-of-fact, but, it's a great motivator, and I kind of wish I'd done this years ago. Stan, my oldest friend and business partner, had agreed to come onboard with me and put some money in as well. We want to extend our reach beyond Liverpool, and help as many people as we can, across the country. Sadly, there will always be homeless people, so Frank 'n' Stan's food vouchers will be a way to get targeted help to those that need it. Me and Stan are not the youngest and have a business to run, so what we wanted to do was start the movement, and have someone younger, with passion, who could help us deliver on our objectives. Which is why we wanted to work with Lee.

Scarlett: Lee, if I can come to you? For those not familiar, you were recently homeless yourself?

Lee looked smart. He was similar height to Frank, so he'd borrowed one of Frank's formal white shirts and a pair of black trousers. Clearly nervous, he cleared his throat before speaking.

Lee: I'm still technically homeless, although Frank and Stan have been good to me and helped me to get on my feet.

Scarlett: Do you mind if I ask how you ended up living on the streets?

Lee paused for a moment and bowed his head, before continuing.

Lee: I had a few problems, back home in Ireland, and tried to make a new life for myself. I came to Liverpool and met a girl, but that didn't work out. Look, I could sit here and fill you with a hard-luck story, but I'd rather look forward than backwards. I met Frank and Stan and loved what they're trying to do. I've promised them that I'll put everything I have into this initiative and I've got a unique perspective in that I've been amongst those we're trying to help.

Scarlett: Frank, if I can come back to you. You're putting some money into this, but how can people help?

Frank: Being homeless is a situation that any of our friends or family could end up in. Like most things, we need money to make this project happen. We've put money in, but we need to fundraise to help as many as we can and that's where Lee is going to add real value, working with homeless charities, and getting out into the community to raise funds. We've got the largest taxi company in the city, so can hopefully offer employment to those who want to get themselves off the streets. It would be great if other employers would work with those who are looking to get into employment. We're new to this, and will learn along the way, but we've got a desire to help and we're all looking forward to the challenge. Lee's passion is going to be crucial in this, but both Stan and I are custodians to make this happen.

Scarlett: Fantastic, and I'm sure you will. And with that, Sally, it's back to the studio to you.

Scarlett's face remained unmoving, as if a PAUSE button had been pressed, until she received the nod from the cameraman that they were no longer live.

"Great, really great work you're doing here, guys," she said warmly, her face reanimated.

Stan had just opened the blind to the small window which separated the two rooms, and Scarlett stared uneasily at it.

"There's a woman... I think... doing something rude at the window," Scarlett said, moving to a position of cover behind the cameraman.

Stella was stood fag in mouth, with a two-finger salute pressed up against the window pane. Stan caught a glimpse and quickly closed the blind once more.

"Don't worry about Stella," said Stan.

"So that was a woman?" Scarlett asked.

"Ostensibly," Stan said.

"It... was horrible," Scarlett said, her face ashen. "It was like bits and pieces cobbled together to form a whole. But not the best bits. Only the worst bits."

Stan laughed. "That's our Stella," he said. "But don't worry. She's just a bit upset she didn't make it onto the interview."

Scarlett laughed nervously and ushered the camera crew to make a hasty exit.

"Thank you, guys, if I can do anything—" she said, calling behind her as she left, before being cut short by the door closing on her way out.

Frank fanned his jumper to get some air to the excessive moisture that'd formed under his armpits.

Lee mopped up a solitary bead of sweat from his temple. "That went okay?" he said in a soft Irish accent.

"That was great," Frank assured him. "But I was shittin' it — it's petty nerve-wracking, ay?"

Lee nodded.

Frank made a furtive glance at the door to make sure Stella was out of earshot.

"Stan, do you honestly think we can leave Stella in charge for two weeks? She's not exactly... y'know... customer-focused?"

"She's not that bad," said Stan.

"She's just told Scarlett Redfern to fuck off!" said Frank.

"It could have been a V for victory?" Stan offered weakly, though he surely knew this hadn't been the case. He chewed his bottom lip for a moment, before continuing, "Yeah, but it's Stella. She'll be alright. Just make sure the bank or anyone important phones us directly. We could see if Lee wants to work from here while we're away... at least he could tell us if the place is falling apart?"

"Where are you guys going?" asked Lee.

"We, as it happens, are going to the TT races," Frank said, his face lit up.

"I went when I was a boy. On the ferry," said Lee. "It's a wonderful place."

"That's not a bad idea," Stan said, responding to Frank's proposition. "Lee, you wouldn't mind working from here for a bit? It'll get you out of that flat during the day?"

"Sure," said Lee. "Cheers. And thank you again for putting me up in your flat, Frank. I can't begin to tell you what it means. If you need me to do anything when you're away, just say the word. I've got a few meetings lined up with the homeless charities and the local paper, so it would be useful to meet them here. In fact, on that subject," said Lee, looking at his watch, "I promised the local school that I'd go in and talk to the ankle-biters about life on the streets."

Lee walked towards the door, but then stopped. He turned and walked back over to Frank and Stan, hugging them each in turn, before leaving without saying another word.

"I think we've done well to find him," said Frank.

Stan did not immediately answer, and Frank turned to him.

"What do you reckon? You don't look convinced, Stan?"

Stan sat on the corner of his desk, arms across his chest, with one hand up to his face, thumb hooked under his chin and forefinger curled like a question mark against his lips.

"I like the guy, don't get me wrong," Stan said. "There's just something... I don't know what. But something I can't quite place my finger on. I'd like to get references. Maybe from a previous employer or landlord?"

"I know," said Frank. "I thought the same. So I've already asked him and he's promised me he'll have something from his previous landlord. He told me he was in the army for a while — a tank driver I think he said — and he's going to have his references sent over. I think we just have to take a leap of faith on him. I've got a good feeling about him."

Stan looked sombre for a moment.

"Frank, I've been putting off asking you this. But are you going to be okay? Y'know. Going away for two weeks?"

Frank shadowboxed for a moment, making a good show of it, but of course Stan couldn't be fooled so easily. Frank knew what he looked like when he peered into the mirror of late, and it wasn't the least bit good.

"I'm fine," said Frank. "In fact it's things like this charity and our bucket list that are keeping me going. I've started the treatment and the doctors seem positive. I know you worry about me, Stan, but don't. The reason I do not want to tell too many people about this is that I don't want them to treat me like a victim. I want them to treat me as, well, like Frank. Just Frank."

"You don't want people to know? You've just been on bloody live television and told the nation!" laughed Stan.

"Oh shit, you're right," said Frank, taking a look at his phone. And sure enough...

"Shit. I've got fifteen missed calls and seven text messages. I suppose I should have told a few people before they heard it whilst eating their breakfast?"

"You reckon?" said Stan, shaking his head and chuckling.

"Ah, well, at least it'll save me having to phone everyone to tell them!" said Frank. "By the way, that Scarlett was a bit of all right, wasn't she!"

"She certainly was, and it's great to see that your libido hasn't been dampened in all of—"

"It'll take more than chemo to dampen my libido!" said Frank, raising himself up proudly. "Ha!"

Stan smiled. "Frank, I don't want to keep asking you how you are, so I won't. But promise me you'll tell me if we're doing too much or if you need to take it easier?"

"I know," said Frank. "And if I don't talk about it, mate, don't think I don't want to share. Maybe it's just the way my brain is wired, but I'm in this situation and just feel talking about it isn't going to change anything. I just want to make the most of the time I've got, and dwelling on it isn't going to help me. Does that make sense?"

"Totally," said Stan. "Anyway, more importantly, who's going to make up with Stella?"

"You think she's mad?" asked Frank.

"Well," said Stan, peering through the window. "Unless I'm very much mistaken, she's currently drawing a huge penis on the back of your coat in black marker pen. So, fortunately, somehow, it would seem, she's just mad with you at the moment!"

chapter eight

the end of May for an avid road racing fan meant only one thing — The Isle of Man TT Races. Held on open roads, it was the ultimate test for the fearless riders who would test their abilities against the 37.73-mile Mountain Course. For two weeks, the small Island in the middle of the Irish Sea became a Mecca for those on two wheels, eager to see their heroes in action or to just marvel at one of the greatest sporting spectacles, anywhere, on earth.

The route for many of those petrol-headed pilgrims was the port of Liverpool, where the Isle of Man's Steam Packet catamaran — *Sea Cat* — would escort them the final eighty or so miles. The vessel sat majestically next to the imposing Royal Liver Building, which was almost as old as the races itself.

The ferry terminal was bursting at the seams with foot passengers urging the call to commence boarding. There were fresh-faced newcomers, who'd avidly watched internet footage and DVDs of the action, but were salivating at the prospect of watching the leading bike head down the daunting Bray Hill on the first day of practice.

Seasoned veterans were also returning, and happy to share anecdotes of the sport they loved with those experiencing it for the first time.

A separate queue formed on the main concourse, where those lucky enough to secure a ticket for their bike would wait with the same sense of exhilaration.

Frank and Stan waited patiently inside the terminal building, absorbing every aspect of the electric atmosphere. The TT Crowd were an eclectic mix covering every spectrum. Some sat on uncomfortable plastic seats, while others congregated on the floor, but regardless of age or nationality, there was a knowing amongst them, a knowing that they were all part of something special. Some of the veterans would look at the newcomers with a sense of jealousy, wishing they could have that feeling, of going for the first time, once again, but they knew that the first thing any of them would do when they returned home was to book two weeks' holiday at the end of May and the beginning of June for the following year.

Once you'd been to the first TT, the thought of two weeks on a beach holiday would seem ludicrous. It was an affliction, a craving, something you build your whole year around.

It wasn't just a holiday — you were part of something, a brotherhood, a special club with an insatiable desire to return each year like a homesick salmon. Many were sat in that room after having their imaginations piqued by first-time visitors the year before; such was the magical state of enamourment towards the event that you returned home and tried to relive the experience to the uninitiated.

But even those with the most vivid imagination were ridiculously wide of the mark. You simply had to experience it for yourself.

"I didn't think it'd be this busy," said Stan. "It was only by luck that I got two cancellations for the ferry. I'm starting to think that I should have booked a hotel in advance now."

Frank laughed until he realised Stan was serious. Frank leaned across the foreign visitor — possibly Dutch — who sat between them. "You've not booked us a hotel?" he said through gritted teeth.

Stan shook his head. "No, but I'm sure it'll be fine, yeah? We'll get a hotel when we get there."

The man between them started to laugh. He was dressed head-to-foot in denim, with a black leather waistcoat that was all but covered in TT badges.

"You're going to try and get accommodation when you *get* there?" the man said, continuing to laugh. "You guys are crazy, I love it!"

Stan looked a bit concerned. "So, no chance of a hotel?" he asked the laughing man.

He was slouched comfortably in his seat, but when he sat upright, it was clear this man was huge, and must have been at least 6-foot-10.

The large, laughing man seemed to consider his response — not wishing, perhaps, to discourage two virgins to the sport he loved. "It's like trying to buy a turkey on Christmas Eve," he said, finally. "Hotels are booked up years in advance."

"Oh dear," said Stan.

"Though you should be able to get into a campsite," the man offered.

"A campsite?" said Stan. "Only we haven't got a tent."

The man-mountain continued to laugh to himself. "I guess this is your first visit to the Isle of Man?" he asked.

Frank nodded. "And possibly the last, if we end up sleeping under the stars."

"You like the bikes?" said the denim-clad man in a thick accent.

Frank shrugged his shoulders. "We like the Isle of Man. We used to go when we were younger. We're going back as it's on our bucket list."

The big man let out a belly laugh that caused the entire waiting room to turn and stare.

"*AH-HA-HA!* A fuck-it list! You guys truly are crazy!"

"No, a..." Frank started to say, but the Laughing Dutchman had already left to join the queue, where he continued to laugh to himself further.

Stan left sufficient time to avoid their new friend before joining the long line. His resolve for the trip appeared to be wavering. He was used to the finer things in life, and the thought of a campsite certainly wasn't appealing to him. Frank had known him too long, and knew what he was thinking.

"Stanley," Frank said. "This is another fine mess you've gotten us into."

"May I be frank with you, Frank?" Stan asked Frank.

"Don't think you're going anywhere," Frank replied. "Even if we've got to sleep in a deckchair, we're going to the Isle of Man."

"Bloody hell," was all Stan could say.

The Irish Sea could be cruel at times, but fortunately for Frank and Stan it was as calm as a millpond as Liverpool disappeared from view behind them. The thought of sleeping under the stars seemed rather less unnerving after their third pint of lager.

Dozens of enthusiasts filled the bar area and people spoke of their previous adventures as others listened intently, toasting to the experience that would soon greet them.

"It's all right, this!" said Stan.

"Bloody marvellous," replied Frank, who, not being an avid drinker, was slurring his words slightly. "We should have done this years ago."

Stan held his gaze as he looked at the huge smile on Frank's face, and his eyes began welling up.

"Just, ah... need some fresh air," Stan said, excusing himself to join the crowd of smokers stood on the outside deck at the rear of the ship.

***

Stan was rarely emotional, so was taken by surprise to find a stream of tears running uncontrollably down his face.

"Everything okay?" asked a concerned woman, turning to see who'd joined their smoking ranks.

"Just the wind," said Stan, indicating the wind had made his eyes water. "But thanks."

He moved to the corner of the deck, looking down on the white foam being kicked up as the ship moved gracefully through the water. The thought of Frank leaving him was awful, simply dreadful. He was as close as a brother to him, and they'd shared every major event as they grew up. Being gay in high school, particularly a tough area of Merseyside, was challenging. Stan never forgot that Frank stood with him, not only then, but through every obstacle they'd faced since. This was Frank's darkest hour, and Stan was wracked with guilt that he'd failed his closest friend when he needed him the most. Perhaps it was the alcohol, but the emotion continued, and Stan gently sobbed.

***

"Here we go," said Frank, opening the heavy watertight door. He struggled to negotiate the weight of the door whilst carrying two plastic beakers of lager, which spilt over with the gentle rocking of the ocean.

"I thought you'd come out here for a crafty ciggy?"

Stan turned his back and raised his hands to his face, taking a moment to adjust his hair.

"Everything okay, Stan? Are you just admiring the view?"

Stan cleared his throat and, despite his best efforts, it was evident from the reddening of his eyes that he was upset.

Frank wasn't stupid, and put his arm gently around him. "It'll be okay, Stan. It'll be okay."

Stan bowed his head. "Frank, I love you. You do know that, don't you?"

"I do," said Frank. "And I'm so grateful that I can call you a friend."

They both leaned on the railing, staring vacantly into the brine below for a fair while, before suddenly feeling a firm, large hand clap down on each of their shoulders.

"My crazy, homeless, fuck-it-list friends!" a booming voice said.

Stan tried to move back but with the force of the arm across his back he was going nowhere. The huge chap from the ferry terminal, the Laughing Dutchman, was stood between them. He was bigger than they'd first thought, and wouldn't have looked at all out of place wrestling Sir Roger Moore in a Bond film.

"God, I bloody love this!" he said in a broken English accent. "I live for this shit!" he announced even louder, to all those stood on the small outside deck. He took up his pint, which had been resting on the floor, and drained the full contents effortlessly.

Stan smiled uneasily and took a sip of his own drink.

"Good, good, smile and nod, Stan," Frank thought to himself. *"Let's hope that appeases him and he'll bugger off."*

The Laughing Dutchman, however, did not bugger off. Instead, he took a step closer and extended his hand, which looked like a shovel — a very *large* shovel. "I'm Henk!" he announced. "Henk, from Holland!"

Stan smiled again, but it was clear that Henk was looking for conversation. "That's Frank and I'm Stan," he said, cautiously shaking the man's hand.

"HA-HA-HA!" laughed Henk. It was the loud laugh of a drunken man, and caused everyone to turn and stare.

"Like Frank-and-Stein Monster!" Henk roared with delight, and then raising his arms, moaning, and stomping like the mythical green creature for additional effect.

"Yes, we get that a lot," Stan said politely.

Stan cleared his throat and pulled Frank toward the door.

"Anyhow, Henk, we really need to go..." he said.

"Yes, yes, we should drink!" said Henk enthusiastically.

He'd mistaken their rebuff as an invite, it would seem, following them back inside to the bar, and — due to his sheer mass — Frank and Stan did not feel compelled to correct him.

The bar was heaving with people, but Henk had the ability to create space for himself. People were cautious of him, Frank and Stan observed, but within ten seconds or so, his laugh — which initially one might find annoying — would have people instantly warmed. What was at first assumed to be intoxication was actually his natural enthusiasm.

People congregated around him, and he told a story like no man they'd ever met. He spoke of his visits to the TT races with such energy that all those stood near to him were arching their necks to listen in, and after he'd finished another in a generous string of anecdotes, he put his hand inside his bag.

"Drinks for all my friends!" the Dutchman insisted, handing the barman a pile of banknotes. "Whatever they want!"

Frank caught the tail end of this as he was returning from the loo. He didn't just buy Frank and Stan a drink, but *the entire bar* a drink.

"Is he a bit crazy?" Frank whispered to Stan once back into earshot.

"He may very well be," said Stan. "But he's just invited us to stay with him."

"All three of us at a campsite?" asked Frank. "Just how big is his bloody tent?"

"No, well I presume he's staying in a house," Stan responded.

"You told him no?" asked Frank.

Stan had a look of uncertainty over his face.

"I'm not sure, to be honest. He offered, started laughing, as he always does, and patted me on the back. We'll just smile politely? Besides, he's been drinking all the way, so he won't even remember us when we get off, most likely," Stan said. "Oh. Hang on. Here he comes."

"You stay with me, my friends from Liverpool. I'll show you the TT!" Henk said, pointing at them both. "Only one bed, it will be cosy!"

Frank was starting to get worried. "Stan," he said out of the corner of his mouth. "Does this big lummox think we're sharing a bed with him for a fortnight?"

Stan started to laugh. "If the big fella said you were sharing a bed with him, you'd be sharing a bed with him! No, what he said when you were powdering your nose is that he has one spare bedroom in a house he's staying at, as two of his friends couldn't make it and he didn't have time to fill it."

"Nice offer," said Frank. "But I think I'd feel more comfortable, and safer, in a hotel. He seems a little... I dunno... unhinged?"

Frank and Stan, like many others, pressed their noses up against the window as the ship eased into the harbour. It'd been years since their last visit, but the memories came flooding back as they were greeted by the Tower of Refuge in Douglas Bay — built to provide safety to stricken mariners since 1832.

They'd exchanged pleasantries with Henk and apprehensively taken his phone number on the pretext of meeting up for a drink at a later date.

"We should have taken him up on his offer," said Stan. "He even offered us a lift with his friend."

"We'll be fine," said Frank. "A chap told me about a snoozebox up at the grandstand, something like a temporary hotel. We'll get a taxi up there, have a look about, couple of pints, and sort a room out. You'll thank me when you find out that Henk is wanted by Interpol."

They stood outside the ferry terminal and waited in line for a taxi, watching as those passengers with bikes made their way onto the Manx roads. The display of a convoy of motorbikes was matched only by the noise they made; it was simply staggering. Locals waved to the new arrivals and received a friendly hoot on the horn as they powered off on the start of their holiday. The atmosphere was electric. The noise of the bikes wasn't just coming from where they stood; there was the constant hum of engines that floated on the breeze.

Frank and Stan were like excitable children as the taxi driver took them along the main promenade, past the famous Bushy's beer tent. Music boomed from the fairground on the seaward side of the road and row upon row of motorbikes were parked up on both sides, stood like dominoes as far as the eye could see. The hair stood up on the back of their necks. The Island was bouncing.

"Are the practices on tonight?" asked Frank of the driver.

"No," replied the cabbie, handing them a small visitors' guide. "No practices on a Sunday. The first one was last night, then every teatime until next Saturday. Then the races are Saturday, Monday, Wednesday, and then the big race is on the Friday. It's all in the guide. It'll be good to have a look around the grandstand — there'll be plenty of people milling about and you should get a pint or two up there."

"We're hoping to get a room in the snoozebox hotel," said Stan.

The taxi driver gave him a look in the rear-view mirror that meant a reservation was anything but likely. "No chance!" he said. "Best chance is a campsite."

"You're not the first to tell us that!" said Frank, glaring at Stan as he did so.

Like many others, the Grandstand was one of the first destinations for those on their TT debut. The pit lane and the scoreboard opposite were iconic — like centre court at

Wimbledon, or the Hôtel de Paris at the Monaco Grand Prix. The park area at the rear was home to the riders and their pit crew for the next two weeks. It was a carnival atmosphere and gave the eager visitor a unique opportunity to walk among their sporting heroes, and observe their teams working on their bikes.

Pop-up shops selling a huge array of motorsport merchandise waited eagerly to lighten the wallets of those looking for a memento of their visit. Elaborate, state-of-the-art race trucks sat proudly near to *parc fermé* — the area where racers would converge before tackling the Mountain Course. The further down the paddock you ventured is where you'd find those without factory funding — the real back-of-your-van racers — for whom the sport was a passion, usually without financial reward. For these riders, the TT was an all-consuming, adrenaline-fuelled adventure that would be funded by themselves and a few generous sponsors. The contrast between the top of the paddock and the bottom was stark, although everyone shared the all-consuming desire to ride out onto the start line on Glencrutchery Road.

The mouth-watering aroma of cooked meat lured Frank and Stan through the busy crowds. Stan's face blushed for a moment as Frank caught him smiling at a tattooed biker.

"You must be like a dog in a butcher's shop with all these men walking around in leather pants!" laughed Frank.

"I hadn't noticed," smirked Stan, and then, "Ah. This must be the Snoozebox Hotel," he said in reference to a towering, portable structure. "It's a bit smaller than I thought."

Any hopes of a room for the night were dashed by a large NO VACANCIES signed placed strategically on several posts driven into the sod.

Frank shook his head. "Shit. Now what?"

Ever the optimist, Stan linked his arm, and said, "We, my good friend, head over to that impressively-appointed beer tent, and have a pint or two of their finest ales just after we have a big, juicy cheeseburger."

"It's not too good for my waistline," said Frank.

Stan rolled his eyes. "Ah, you'll be dead soon anyways. Live a little!"

Two pints turned to three as they soaked up both the atmosphere of the paddock and the brew in their cups.

"If it's like this in practice week, imagine what it's going to be like in race week!" said Stan as they reluctantly, and slightly unsteadily, wandered through the maze of trucks, vans, and tents.

"We'll need to walk down to the promenade and see if they have any cancellations?" suggested Frank.

It was early evening, and from every van or awning they walked by came a sound of tinkering: the noise of ratchets and wrenches bouncing on metal, as intense mechanics stooped over their vehicles to make alterations — anything they could do to drag an extra horsepower out of their finely-tuned engines. Lower down the paddock, riders were genuinely pleased if you took a moment to pop your nose into their temporary garage, and would happily talk you through their racing career, or the motivation that brought them to the Island. The thing they all had, every one of them, was a passion. Their eyes widened as they spoke about their sport, and it was infectious.

Even though they'd already eaten, Frank and Stan were offered the spoils of a BBQ each time they stopped to speak to another outfit, and another beer was thrust into their hands.

At the end of a row of vans, they came upon an awning with a shabby, oil-stained leather couch underneath that looked like it'd been found abandoned by a canal. It was positioned facing in, with only its back clearly visible. Tucked beside the couch was something unusual. All Frank and Stan had seen so far had been motorbikes. When they clapped eyes on Sidecar Number 42, however, they beheld a thing of beauty.

"Look at that!" said Stan shrilly, his voice rising several octaves. "That's amazing!"

The shell of this magnificent device glistened as the remains of the day's sun bounced off its immaculate paintwork. The colour scheme was like something from a psychedelic dream — blue & yellow — which made it look like a giant boiled sweet.

As they walked closer, Stan pulled his phone out of his pocket to take a picture. As he approached, the sudden, deafening noise of metal clanging against metal gave him quite a start, and caused him to pull back, curling his phone up to his chest.

"You useless piece of shit!" screamed a disembodied voice.

Frank, either brave or foolhardy, walked cautiously and peered into the workshop behind the sidecar. A crazed-looking brute of a man stood staring, with demonic eyes, at the machinery before him. He held a spanner that was the length of a baby's arm, and he swayed back and forth like he was preparing to attack. He must have sensed he was being watched, because suddenly his head turned.

Frank had been spotted. He froze.

The man was tensed up, like a coiled spring. He stood barefoot, wearing only a pair of oil-stained white Y-fronts and a t-shirt with FRANKIE SAYS RELAX on the front. The shirt was at least a couple of sizes too small, and the man's belly broke free of its constraints, poking out in a large bulge between it and the underpants, giving the appearance of a sausage that'd been tied too tightly around the middle. Fragments of an engine lay strewn about, and the spanner in the man's hand was the likely cause of the sporadic dints on the engine itself, listing sadly to one side on a workbench. It looked very much like various engine parts, impossibly, had been separated from the main by vicious whacks of the spanner.

In the blink of an eye, the brute was upon them, arm extended, massive, beastly paw at the ready with what could only be considered ill-intent.

Frank and Stan cringed, eyes shut tightly, waiting for the rain of blows...

...which never came. "I'm Dave!" said Dave.

Tightly-clenched eyes opened, cautiously. They beheld a wide grin, and a hand, quite innocently, held out for a shake.

"Sorry about the ruckus! Engine trouble!" said Dave amiably, as he shook Stan and Frank's hands in turn.

"Self-inflicted, judging by the dints?" Frank ventured. "I wasn't sure whether we should call for security."

"Ha-ha! Was I making that much noise?" said Dave.

"No," said Frank. "I meant more for the dress sense."

Dave's face turned serious and he took a step forward. He was over 6 ft tall and built like the side of a house. He dropped the spanner and extended his arms, causing Frank to shrink back into his shell like a startled hermit crab, certain he'd finally gone too far, and braced himself again for the worst.

Again, the worst never came.

"I like you!" said Dave, gathering them up and ushering them inside. He reached inside a beer fridge, which had a dangerous amount of electrical cables running into it.

"Beer!" Dave cried out, several bottles now in hand. It was rather more an exclamation than a question.

Frank didn't want to offend him twice, considering the huge spanner was within clubbing distance. "Yeah... sure," Frank said slowly and carefully, not wishing to cause upset. "Anything we can do to help?" he added.

The extent of Frank's mechanical knowledge could be written on the back of a postage stamp in thick black marker pen, as Stan well knew.

"And what exactly are you going to do with that engine?" laughed Stan, who was now also in receipt of a cold beer.

Frank shrugged his shoulders. "Not much. Only I felt quite manly being in a garage with all the dirt and tools, didn't I? And I thought it was the right thing to say besides."

"You calling me a tool??" demanded Dave.

"What? No! I meant..." stuttered Frank.

Dave gave him a friendly slap on the back that nearly launched him off his feet.

"You could help me if you've got a race-tuned engine for a Suzuki GSX-R600 in your hand luggage!" laughed Dave.

"Is this engine knackered, then?" asked Frank.

Dave looked disapprovingly at the mauled carcass sat on the bench.

"If it was a dog, we'd put it down," he said bluntly.

"Ah!" said Frank, maintaining his manly interest. "What happened?"

"I've dropped a valve," said Dave matter-of-factly.

Frank sniffed the air and took a step back, scanning the floor for the valve gone missing.

"On the bike!" explained Dave. "Engines don't like a dropped valve."

"Have you not got a spare?" asked Stan.

"Yes," said Dave. "Can you give me a hand getting it? It's wrapped in cashmere in the back of my gold-plated Lamborghini."

"Ah," said Stan. "I take it they're expensive?"

Dave nodded his head in resignation, "Four thousand, maybe as much as six, at this late stage. That's on top of the twenty thousand I've spent on the bike itself. The joys of racing! Still, I've got two weeks off work and the beer fridge is well stocked. So it's not all bad news, I suppose."

"So, you can't race?" asked Frank.

"No. The only way I'd get that bike around the TT course is if I cut two holes in the bottom and run around, Fred Flintstone-style."

"I'm very sorry to hear that," said Stan. "Do you not have any sponsors?"

Before Dave had a chance to reply, Frank stepped forward and took a large mouthful of beer. His mouth now well-lubricated, out came this:

"If we buy you a new engine, can we put the name of our charity on the sidecar?"

Dave laughed. "If you buy me a new engine, you can tattoo the name of your charity on both my arse cheeks. I'm being serious."

Stan smiled. "That's a great idea. I mean the engine. Not the tattoo. Although..."

"Hang on. Are you two taking the piss?" asked Dave.

"No," replied Frank. "We're deadly serious. Call it a whim, senility, an impulse, or whatever."

"Or whatever," Stan agreed.

"But it'd be amazing to be part of a race team," Frank continued. "We've just started a charity and it'd be a really good way of advertising what it does."

"A good way," Stan chimed in.

"What does it do?" asked Dave, barely able to contain himself.

"We give food stamps to the homeless," Stan and Frank said in unison.

Dave's eyes drifted down to his stomach, and then back up at them.

"You want *me* to be a poster boy for the hungry?"

"Yes," replied Frank. "The publicity would be good, and you can teach me a thing or two about mechanics?"

"Monty is going to be over the moon," declared Dave.

Stan looked around.

"Who's Monty?"

"Shaun Montgomery, my sidecar passenger," said Dave by way of explanation, but was met only by looks of confusion from Frank and Stan. "Monty, wake up!" shouted Dave, throwing a small metal bolt past them.

Stan and Frank had been with their backs to the oil-stained couch, and had given it no attention at all since they'd first encountered it, and were thus startled to see a cross-eyed man, roused from slumber, rise slowly from its depths, still clutching a can of beer.

It turnt out there'd been life couched within that couch the whole time.

"He didn't take the news about our retirement well," said Dave, in reference to the array of crushed cans spread over the grass like jetsam thrown out a boat and washed ashore.

Monty wiped the crust from his eyes and blinked.

"Monty, my old son, you're going to have to squeeze into those leathers after all! Because of these two crackpots, the team is back in business! We've got ourselves a sponsor — Frank 'n' Stan's Food Stamps!"

Bear hugs were then given by Dave, from which Frank and Stan fruitlessly struggled to escape.

"You just sort the engine out, Dave, and tell us where to send the cash," Frank said. "Look, not be rude but we need to be on our way, actually. We've only arrived just today, and we need to find a hotel."

Dave looked like he was about to drop another valve.

"The team principals do not stay in a hotel. No, they do not. Not a chance! Monty, get the guest quarters prepared, we've got visitors staying with us!"

"Wait, we've got an engine?" Monty said drowsily, rubbing his eyes again to get the sleepybugs out of them, leaving a smear of black grease over his face in the process.

"That we have, Monty. That we have," said Dave. "We're going racing, baby!"

The paddock was alive early and the sound of revving engines meant a long lie in bed was all but impossible. Not that a long lie-in would have been desirable anyway, as Dave's definition of getting the guest quarters prepared was slightly different to what Frank and Stan had imagined.

"Morning, teammates!" said Dave enthusiastically. "Did you sleep okay?"

Dave lay back on the mattress, arms stretched out across the width of it, with Frank cushioned into one of his armpits and Stan into the other. Despite the circumstance, his excited smile remained infectious.

"Sorry for the smell, chaps, but I wasn't expecting any company other than Monty, and sleeping in the back of a transit van doesn't give you the best of showering facilities."

"It's fine," said Stan graciously. "But I do feel a bit guilty about throwing Monty out of his bed. Is that couch comfortable?"

"He'll be fine on that couch."

"Thinking about it," said Stan. "You both live over here, so what are you doing sleeping in the back of your van?"

"Because I love it," Dave said. "I love every aspect of the fortnight — the smells, the noise, the atmosphere, the comradery. I love everything about it and if I sleep at home I feel like I'm missing out on something. Monty's the same, he can't get enough of it, either."

"Look, Dave," said Frank. "It's really generous of you to put us up last night. But I don't think the three of us can sleep in the back of your van another night. We'll try and get a hotel sorted, if you don't mind. Just so you know, and I know we'd had a few beers on board, but I'm deadly serious about the engine."

Dave jumped up. "Fantastic! If I can get me some logos from your website or something, I'll get the printers to sort the stickers out."

"Can we put one on your helmet?" asked Stan.

"Oo-er, Matron, you won't see it for my trousers. Not a problem, I'll get that sorted," Dave said. "If you don't mind, gents," he continued, "I'm going to get on. I need to source the engine, and see if we can get the bike up to the test track in Jurby to give her a run out. Take my phone number, and if you need anything while you're here, just let me know? The practices are on tonight and if you want to come up here to the pits and watch, you can help the guys with refuelling, or, I'll give you a fantastic spot to watch from. We're going to get to a hundred and five miles per hour this time. I can feel it in my water!"

"A hundred and five miles per hour?" asked Stan, very underwhelmed. "I've done that in my taxi going up the M6."

"I like your spunk!" said Dave. "That's the average speed over the entire length of the course, though. You wouldn't be doing that in your taxi, not unless it had wings!"

Monty appeared, clutching sausage baps. He was an interesting character; his passion and zeal were immediately apparent, and Frank and Stan warmed to him instantly. Like Dave, it was evident from their generous waistlines that they weren't natural athletes, but what they lacked in sporting prowess they made up for in gusto.

The thought of staying in the back of a transit van was far from appealing the night before, but within half an hour in their company, listening to their stories of previous TTs, they got it, they understood, and sleeping on a couch in the middle of a field made perfect sense.

Frank and Stan left their bags with Dave and walked down to Douglas Promenade, covered in the stale aroma that came from three men sharing a bed for the evening.

"I've got an idea," said Stan, placing his phone to his ear.

"Yes, hello, Stella? Stella, its Stan."

He struggled to hear as the sound of a passing bike thundered in front of him. "Stella, it's Stan, can you hear me?"

He nodded his head before turning to Frank, "We're dickheads, apparently." And, back to Stella, "Thanks for that, Stella. What've we done wrong, then? Well, what's Lee done wrong?"

He continued to nod. "Okay, well, that's good. That's what we wanted him to do... I know the office isn't a soddin' drop-in centre. Stella, listen, I don't have a lot of charge left on my phone. Me and Frank are struggling to get a hotel. We need you to phone a few and see if you can get us a reservation. We're going to walk round a few but it'll be quicker if you can phone? Okay, great, aha... Thanks, Stella."

"Sorted?" asked Frank.

Stan smiled. "She said she's not our fucking secretary, so no, not sorted. Remind me why we employ her again?"

"Great. And what's Lee done to annoy her?" asked Frank.

"Nothing. He's had people dropping clothes off at the office to give out to the homeless. And he's given a collection bucket to every driver on the night shift. He raised over fourteen-hundred quid last night!"

"What! That's amazing!"

Frank looked concerned as they continued walking along the promenade.

"There's not quite as many hotels as I remember. It looks like there are more apartment blocks now. I don't think this is going to be a success, judging by the no vacancies signs in the windows. I'm starting to think we need to—"

"Phone the crazy Dutch bloke?" interrupted Stan.

"It's either that or another night in the back of the transit van, with Dave's underarms for pillows."

"I'm ringing Henk now!"

chapter nine

monty was, without doubt, the most enthusiastic co-pilot a man could wish for. He'd taken to racing later in life than most, and it could be argued he wasn't the best there was. But he wasn't just about the glory of turning up to race; he was the man who was committed all year round. It was only his second year racing with Dave, but he was always as excited as a dog eating chips. Nothing was a chore and every task was met with complete commitment.

"There's good and bad news," declared Monty.

Dave popped his head from under the sidecar. "You've found a page-three model, but she's only got eyes for me?"

"No, well, not yet," Monty said, wiping the sweat from his forehead. "I've just found us an engine!"

Dave jumped up. "That's amazing! Well done! Why's that bad news? The cost?"

"I don't know about the cost. But it belongs to the McMullan brothers. Tom's fractured wrist hadn't healed as well as they thought, as it turns out, and he's had to pull out of the race."

"Fuck. Well, that's that, then. I'm not going cap-in-hand to them couple of arseholes. I'll just get on the phone and see if I can get a standard engine."

"Dave, it may have escaped your notice, but we're not exactly the slimmest guys on the paddock. We need every horsepower we can get hold of. Otherwise it'll be as slow as driving in treacle."

"Or Lyle's Golden Syrup," Dave said dreamily.

"Dave! Snap out of it! We need their engine!"

Dave crossed his arms and caressed the two-day growth on his chin. They'd both worked all year for this; pride was telling him to forget it, but deep down, he knew it was the only opportunity to race. If they had a standard engine, it'd be that slow carrying the pair of them that they'd have no chance of getting a qualifying time to race.

"Aw, bollocks. Okay, I'll do it. I don't like it. But I'll do it."

Monty slapped him on the back, "Just focus on the hundred-and-five miles per hour, Dave. Just focus."

The McMullan brothers had funding, and with that came the best of everything: motorhome, equipment, leathers, you name it, they had it. They were talented, all right, but just thoroughly repugnant. Dave marched across the paddock, rehearsing what he was going to say. His inner voice was calm and conciliatory, but as soon as he clapped eyes on Tom or Harry, he knew he'd have to resist the urge to stick a torque wrench where it didn't belong.

As he walked along, Dave gained some small satisfaction by considering the correct application of the wrench, working out just how many ft-lbs of pressure might be applied.

Harry McMullan sat under his canopy looking forlorn. A stream of fans waited patiently to get a programme signed or a photograph with him. He wasn't interested, and his signature in their prized possession was nothing but a scrawl. Dave waited patiently as the small queue dispersed. Harry signed the last programme and looked up at Dave.

"You want a photograph with me?" said McMullan, pretending not to recognise him, and then, "Oh. Apologies. Are you here to empty the chemical toilet?"

A hundred and eighty foot-pounds, Dave thought. A hundred and eighty should be about right.

"I'm sorry to hear about your brother, Harry," Dave managed diplomatically. "I understand he cannot drive, because of his wrist?"

McMullan didn't respond; he just sat scraping oily grime from under his fingernails with a penknife.

"Harry, I know we've never got on, but—"

"Twenty grand," Harry said without raising his head. "For the engine. Twenty grand and it's yours."

Dave's composure quickly evaporated, "You know what, Harry, you're such a prick. You can stick the engine up your sanctimonious, scrawny arse."

McMullan laughed. "That engine is the best-tuned on the Island, ready to race, and could be in your flea-pit of an awning in ten minutes, good to go out and practice tonight."

"Even if I had that sort of money, I'd rather employ a hitman than give it you."

"Fine, should I tell my brother you were asking after him?"

"No," said Dave. "I've got a funny feeling you're going to be joining him in the fracture clinic, though."

"Temper, temper!"

Dave turned his back on him. "Oh, do you know what? Stick it. You and your dopey brother can kiss my hairy Manx arse."

Harry let him walk to the entrance before standing theatrically.

"Okay, okay, out of respect for a fellow racer, I'll do you a deal."

Dave wanted to carry on walking, but had to listen to what McMullan might have to say. He stopped, but didn't turn round.

"Go on, then."

"Dave, for you, I'm going to let you have the engine for the princely sum of... one pound."

Dave looked over his shoulder, fists clenched, certain McMullan was taking the piss, and he did not fancy being made a fool of.

The look in Dave's eyes was one of dire enmity. Harry was arrogant, but knew if Dave hit him, he'd wake up at the end of the week. "Ah, temper, Dave," he said, raising his hands in submission. "I'm being deadly serious now. The engine is yours. No charge."

Dave turned to face McMullan. He was irritated, but needed to see where this was heading.

"Let's not do that thing they do in films where there is a last-minute demand and an audible exhale of surprise. We both know you want something, so out with it."

"Okay, Dave. As you know, Tom cannot drive because of his wrist, but there's nothing wrong with *me*. Get rid of that Minty fellow and I'll be your passenger."

"It's Monty. And not a hope in hell."

"Dave, don't be an idiot. I'm the best passenger you could have, and you'd have the best engine. You could get a hundred-and-ten-mile-per-hour lap, no problem."

Harry stepped closer. "Dave, I'm being deadly serious here. I've met Monty. He's a nice enough bloke, but come on, he's not a very good passenger and you know it. This is a once-in-a-lifetime opportunity. You will never get the chance to have this package again. Monty would understand, if he's a friend, he'd never let you pass up on this opportunity."

Dave stood silent. But he was still listening.

"Dave, you're, what, early forties? This is your last chance to compete at this level. Don't let your pride get in the way of this opportunity. This is everything you've ever wanted."

Harry McMullen took a chance, a rather large chance, and stretched up — because it was a stretch — to place both his hands on Dave's shoulders.

"Forget about Monty."

chapter ten

next time, let me arrange the travel bookings?" said Frank, wiping sweat from his face.

"What?" protested Stan. "We've been here a day and the boat was fine, you've had a nice sleep—"

"In the back of a bloody van!"

"You've had a nice sleep," repeated Stan. "The crazy man has offered us accommodation, and now I've arranged us transport. All in all, that's not a bad result, I would say. Now stop your bloody whinging and carry on pedalling."

"I'm not a well man," continued Frank. "I'm on my last legs and you've got my legs out cycling."

"Stop being so melodramatic, Frank. A bit of gentle exercise will do you good, besides, and that's why I've gotten us a tandem bike."

"I still need to pedal, though, Stan, and I've not showered for some time, so my personal hygiene would, at best, be considered questionable. This is not helping."

"Hardly peddling — it's an electric bike. Every car was booked out, so this is the next best thing. Can you have a look at the maps on your phone and see where Henk's house is?"

"Already done. I'll give you directions, but I don't have much life left in my phone so we'll need to be fairly quick — turn that electric engine up to maximum."

With the battery on the bike it was like having the benefit of a prevailing wind providing a gentle push along, and Frank's scepticism was soon replaced with a huge smile. It'd been years since he'd been on a bike.

Broadway was a challenging incline which led from Douglas Promenade all the way up to the top of Bray Hill, a short distance from the Grandstand, but with modern technology and two pairs of legs, they made short work of it. The house was in the general direction of the Grandstand, and from where they'd just come from.

"That dog is looking a bit too interested in us!" shouted Stan in between several heavy breaths.

An ugly dog with a face like it'd been hit with a spade was jogging parallel to them, on the pavement. They were at the steepest part of the hill, but, Stan, spurred on by being stalked like prey, found a final burst of energy and increased speed.

"Come on, Frank, put some effort in," he said as he pressed frantically on the control panel of the bike, trying to draw a further burst from the battery.

The dog kept pace without breaking sweat, and it started to increase its canter as it jumped from the pavement and onto the road.

"Shit!" shouted Frank. "It's directly behind us now! And it doesn't look too happy! Wait, no, it's hard to tell with that mashed-in face..."

"Well is it happy or unhappy?" Stan asked desperately.

"Yeah, no, it's started to growl. So definitely unhappy, I'd say."

Stan gave it everything and they were soon doing a pace that Bradley Wiggins would be proud of. Even so...

"It's not good, Stan!" Frank warned. "It's gaining on us."

"Kick the little bastard!" shouted Stan.

"I'm bloody pedalling! How can I kick it?"

Stan arched his neck and the bike wobbled unsteadily.

"I feel like a bloody gazelle on the Serengeti being stalked by a malnourished lion!" said Stan.

"Only not a gazelle," Frank offered. "Maybe more like a water buffalo?"

"Do something, Frank! Throw something at it!" shouted Stan with increasing panic. "I bloody hate dogs!"

"What can I throw at it? I haven't gotten anything to throw!" said Frank.

"Do I have to think of everything?" yelled Stan. "Throw your shoe at it!"

"But I need my shoes!" protested Frank. "How else am I going to get about?"

"You'll still have the one! And, besides. If that dog gets hold of your leg, one is all you'll need anyhow as your leg will end up its dinner!"

Frank struggled with his shoe and the momentum of the bike. He'd soon worked it loose and, like a pilot opening the bomb bay doors, he lined up his target with precision. He released the weapon, and it flew directly towards their four-footed pursuer.

The dog lifted its head and gratefully caught Frank's shoe in its maw with ease.

"Well?" shouted Stan.

"It's eating my bloody shoe!" shouted Frank. "But I think it's only made him angrier, there's some sort of white foam running down its face! Look, we're going to have to stop."

"What? That's hardly a good plan, Frank!"

"I'm knackered, I can't pedal anymore!"

With no other option available, they pulled over to the side of the road, with concerned drivers — who'd witnessed the chase — observing the spectacle as they passed by. They were not concerned enough, unfortunately, to stop and render assistance, it would seem.

The dog dropped the shoe and made straight for Stan's waist, where it latched onto his trousers. Frank picked up his shoe — which was covered in puncture wounds and slobber — and started to hit the dog, but to little effect. The dog shook its head furiously, and with minimal resistance, most of Stan's left trouser leg came away and now flapped in the wind from the canine's jaws.

"Little bastard's got my trousers!" screamed Stan.

The dog's focus turned toward the pocket area of what up till very recently had been Stan's trouser leg, and tore at it until a large pork pie fell out and rolled merrily down the hill. The dog turned and ran after it.

"A pork pie!" shouted Frank. "That's what it was after! Why did you let me throw my shoe — which cost two-hundred pounds — when you had a pie in your pocket!"

"I was hungry," said Stan by way of explanation.

"You were hungry! My shoe now has rabies because you were hungry!"

"And it was a gala pork pie," added Stan.

"A gala pork pie?" demanded Frank.

"Yes. The kind with a hard-cooked egg in the middle."

"I know what it is!" Frank shouted.

"They're my favourite," said Stan, shrugging his shoulders, as if this should have been both obvious and explanation enough.

"Look, I didn't come out of this unscathed," Stan continued. "I've lost half of my trousers, after all," he said, looking for signs of injury, of which there were fortunately none. "Come on, we need to go and get our bags back from Dave's, I can't walk around like this, I'll be nicked for indecent exposure."

The dog, at the foot of the hill, was now on its back, bollocks in the air, wriggling about, rubbing itself against the tarmac and making happy grunting noises.

Stan's trousers, or what yet remained of them, flapped like a torn sail as they powered the bike up once more and sped off. It was a godsend — the bike, that is — and, on reflection, quicker to navigate the roads which were congested with traffic.

"We won't get our bags on this thing," said Stan as they cycled, near their destination now, through the crowded paddock. "We'll need to leave the bike, grab the bags, and walk to Henk's house. Are we doing the right thing, Frank? What if he is some sort of nutter? I mean, who invites two complete strangers to stay in their house?"

"I don't think it's his, more of a rental for a couple of weeks, but I take your point. Look, if it doesn't feel right, we'll just turn back round. If we do, I think we're best off heading home, and we can sort something out for next year."

"Bit optimistic?" asked Stan.

"I'm trying to remain positive, Stanley, I have every intention of being above ground next year."

"I meant optimistic about getting a hotel for next year, not pushing up daisies. Although with your illness, it would probably make sense to not pay a deposit. You know, just in case," laughed Stan.

The joke was not lost on Frank, who clipped Stan across the back of the head.

Monty laid on the grubby couch with a dirty cloth covering his face. He said nothing, apart from a periodic expletive, and did nothing apart from kicking the arm of the couch with his heel.

Frank and Stan were surprised to see a scene of relative quiet, as opposed to last-minute race preparations, and parked up their bike.

"Everything okay, guys?" said Frank.

Monty didn't move.

"Did you get your hotel sorted?" asked Dave, stepping out of his van. "Nice tandem, by the way!"

Stan shook his head. "No, as they'd say in the bible, no room at the inn. We're going to hopefully stay with the chap we met on the boat, so just needed to grab our bags," he said, and then added, "Is Monty alright?"

Dave's jolly demeanour dropped as Monty sat upright.

"I'm fine," said Monty, his voice raw. "Twelve months of work down the shitter, that's all."

"I've had to give him some unlucky news," said Dave. "He won't be racing, and, understandably, he's taken it badly."

"What?" said Frank. "That's awful, sorry to hear it. What happened?"

Dave took up his customary pose of arms crossed, rubbing his chin. He took a deep breath. "No engines. Anywhere. I could get a second-hand, bog-standard one, but it's pointless. So, sadly, without a race-tuned engine, we're calling it a day. If you're coming back over next year, we'd love it if you wanted to sponsor us then?"

Frank slapped him on the side of the arm. "Sorry, mate. At least this means you can join us for a pint or two?"

"Lead the way, my friend," replied Dave.

"We need to go and check this house out first," said Stan.

"And showered," said Dave, turning his nose up.

"Yes, and showered. Come on, Frank, Henk said if we can get to him before four, he'll show us around and give us a spare key. We can check to see if there are any dead bodies lying around."

"Henk?" asked Dave.

Stan nodded. "Henk! This slightly eccentric fellow we met on the boat. He's from Holland."

"Fuck off!" said Dave.

Stan looked at Frank. "Bit harsh?"

"Dutch Henk? About seven-foot tall?" asked Dave.

"Yes," Stan said. "The Laughing Dutchman, we call him." And then, hesitantly, "How, erm, do you know him, exactly? Is he completely mental?"

Dave laughed. "Very possibly. The guy is an absolute legend. He's been coming to the TT for years. He's absolutely loaded, owns car and motorbike dealerships all over Europe. He sponsors a few of the top riders. I was at a party he was at a few years ago and the guy is completely crazy — I've never seen anyone drink like that boy!"

"Hmm," was all Stan replied.

"Stan, you know I'm not one for fashion," added Dave. "But what the hell is going on with those trousers?"

"Long story, involving a hungry mutt. Can we lock our bike up, here? At least till we drop the bags off?"

"Sure," said Dave. "But don't leave it too long. There's no point in us leaving our stuff down here, as we're going to pack our stuff up and head home soon. Sadly, our TT dream is over for the year."

"You still here?" came a jovial, smug voice from two awnings up. "In case you were worried about me, don't. I've got a ride with Tony Dearie."

"Who's that plonker?" whispered Stan. "Friend of yours, Dave?"

"Not hardly," Dave replied. "That's Harry McMullan. Good racer, but a complete WOMBLE!" And he said *womble* loud enough so that McMullan was certain to hear it well enough.

Monty raised his head. "Micky Fitzpatrick's racing with Tony Dearie. Is he alright?"

"He's fine, Minty!" McMullan called over.

"It's Monty! You stupid git!" shouted Dave. "MONTY. It's not that hard!"

McMullan only feigned offence. "I'll tell you what else wasn't hard," he said. "Was Tony Dearie deciding he didn't want to be a loser, like you two. Tony's parted company with Micky, and is now in possession of one of the quickest engines on the grid. Something you'd have had, Dave, if you weren't so stupid."

Dave glared daggers over at McMullan, but McMullan continued on, undaunted. "Look at you, stood there with your knuckles virtually dragging on the ground. And Monty there. I mean, seriously? You could have been racing with *me*, but you chose him instead. He's got one eye looking *at* me and the other looking *for* me — how does he even know which bend to aim for? Those two gawkers," McMullan said, pointing to Frank and Stan, "Would jolly well be more competitive on their little two-wheeled tandem than you two overweight Neanderthals. Be sure to give me a little wave when you've packed your van up. I might even park mine on your pitch."

"A real charmer, he is," said Stan,

Dave raised his chubby middle finger and threw it in McMullan's direction. "Isn't he just!"

Monty padded over quietly, unable to raise his head. "You could have had his engine, and him as a passenger, but you refused?" he asked Dave.

"I refused because he's a complete cock. If he was alright I'd be helping you pack your bags myself, Monty."

"I know you don't mean that, Dave, but for what it's worth, thank you."

"Christ almighty," said Dave. "If we were in a film, some dodgy Celine Dion track would now be playing as we both look lovingly into each other's eyes."

This got a laugh out of Monty.

"I race because I want to race," Dave continued on. "There's no chance I'm ever going to be on the top step at the garlanding ceremony. I might get a few extra miles per hour out of his engine, sure. But ultimately, I want to enjoy it. I enjoy riding with *you*, Monty. The only way I'd enjoy riding with *him* is if I were in my car and it was over his leg."

Monty smiled and tucked his head into Dave's bosom as he started singing — very badly — "My Heart Will Go On" by Celine Dion.

chapter eleven

like most who've been invited to stay with a friend, there's always that nagging doubt as to whether the polite invite was genuine or merely rhetorical.

"My fuck-it friends!" Henk shouted on his doorstep at their arrival, his deep, booming voice both clearing the fog for a several-mile radius and frightening the sheep.

An epic bearhug from Henk, accompanied by deep belly laugh, were enough to allay any fears that Frank and Stan may have had.

"Please, come in, make yourself at home," Henk offered. "You should shower!" he added, though his intentions there were likely not entirely altruistic.

Frank and Stan hadn't had a wash since they'd left Liverpool and, since, had slept in a van using a man's hairy underarms as pillows and been chased down by a crazed dog, amongst other misadventures. In short, they stank.

"Stan," enquired Henk. "You do know you have only one trouser leg?"

"It's a long story," Stan said. "Perhaps best told later on over several beers."

"Ah. Well in that case, come, I'll show you to your room for now," Henk said.

"Henk," Stan began, "Can I just say, thank you for—"

"After which, you can take a shower!" Henk continued.

"You've really helped us out, Henk," Stan carried on. "We really do appreciate it. We couldn't find anywhere to stay. We slept in a sidecar racer's van last night, nestled under his armpits, as it happens..."

"You'd probably like to shower!" Henk suggested.

"It's a lovely place you've got here," said Stan, admiring the house. "Is this yours?"

"This is my home-away-from-home on the Isle of Man. I rented it for years, but, since I intend to retire here on the Island anyway, I ended up simply buying the house."

"Close to the TT course, as well," said Frank.

The property was similar to Franks, sat at the end of a private driveway with a few other properties, but this was huge. Really huge.

Frank looked over Henk's shoulder. Or around his shoulder, at least, since looking over Henk's shoulder was not easily accomplished. "Is, eh, that a swimming pool you've got there, Henk?" he asked.

"Always a good idea to take a quick shower before jumping in a pool!" Henk said as a bit of useful trivia.

In the marble-floored entrance hall were several racing bikes, with pictures displayed along the walls of Henk stood with rider after rider. Frank wasn't the most clued up about racers, so avoided the embarrassment of asking who they were. He arched his neck to look at the pictures, which continued up along the imposing staircase. In fact, there were motorsport memorabilia everywhere — not just bikes, but cars, sidecars, enduro bikes, and rally cars. It was a petrolhead's dream.

"If you're quick," said Henk, looking at his watch, "I'll take you to my favourite viewing spot to watch the practice session. You'll love it. Meet you downstairs in twenty minutes. Feel free to take a shower!"

Frank threw his bag on the bed. "This place is freaking amazing," he whispered. "We've landed on our feet with this." Then he said, turning to face Stan, "What do we do about money?"

"For what?" asked Stan.

"For Henk. We can't stay in this place for two weeks without paying for the room?"

"I don't think he needs the cash, but it would be good to offer. Maybe we can take him out for a nice meal or something. You can decide," Stan said, then added, "You outrank me."

"What? I thought we were equal partners?" Frank said, confused.

"No, I meant you jump in the shower first. I smell," Stan explained. "But you *really* smell."

It was difficult to comprehend that the roads they'd only just driven were now closed and become a racing circuit. Handed over to race control each evening for the practice sessions and a large portion of race week, the transformation was remarkable. The logistics to turn this small island in the middle of the Irish Sea into one of the most iconic racing circuits on earth was simply staggering, even more so when you consider the roads had to facilitate the daily commute of the island's residents a short while earlier.

The beating pulse at the heart of this operation was an unpaid army of volunteer marshals, known affectionately as the Orange Army due to the colour of their high-vis jackets and vests. They were required to ensure the safety of both the spectators and the racers. To do this effectively, each group of marshals had to maintain a line of sight with the next group; with over 200 corners on a 37.7-mile-long course, it was a challenge.

Henk and two of his friends spoke at a frantic pace, in Dutch, stopping periodically to share a brief translation into English for Stan and Frank's benefit. For two city boys, the walk along the disused Douglas-to-Peel railway line was captivating. Surrounded by rolling Manx countryside, it was easy to close your eyes and imagine the shrill whistle and smells of the steam trains that once served this route.

They were perfectly happy to carry on walking, before Henk ushered them up a side lane. He switched his pocket radio on and the sound of revving engines boomed out of it, disturbing the tranquillity.

"This place will blow you away!" effused Henk, as his friends shared a knowing look. They could speak English, it seemed, but were not as accomplished as their host, who now looked like a child in a toy shop as he quickened his pace.

A quaint white cottage sat at the top of the lane, next to the main road which was now a racetrack. The building had aged gracefully and would have been privy to the evolution of motorsport from its enviable location. A thick piece of rope with an oil-stained flag draped in the middle was all that separated spectators from the racing. On their car journey out, they'd seen hundreds of people crowded on the hedgerows, vying for a prime vantage point, and were surprised that they shared this spot with one tired-looking mountain biker who was mostly covered in dried mud. He also smiled and had the look that something special was about to happen.

The energy level of the radio commentator had reached fever pitch as the first of the bikes left the grandstand for Monday night's practice session. Frank peered over the rope towards the two sets of marshals located at either end of the long stretch of tarmac. As soon as the bikes were en route, the orange-clad volunteers jumped up and were poised to greet the first arrivals.

They were a little over four miles away, where they stood, from the starting point, and the contrast between screaming bikes at the grandstand heard over the radio and calm silence presently at their location was stark. A light breeze ruffled the branches in the trees that lined the road. A chorus of birdsong filled the idyllic countryside, with one particular bird gliding leisurely down to retrieve a discarded snack from the middle of the road.

Henk lowered the volume on his radio to inaudible level and put his finger to his lips, looking over at Frank and Stan expectantly.

Frank strained his face as he caught the distant sound of engines, getting closer by the second. It was strangely compelling, and caused a wave of anxiety to flash through his body, like watching a horror movie and waiting nervously to be startled at any moment. The breeze seemed to amplify the roar of engines hurtling up Ballahutchin Hill, a mile or so from where they stood, the sound of it riding the wind. The marshals leaned forward to maximise their view, and the bird that floated down moments ago instinctively knew it was now time to take flight.

Frank looked over at Stan, who was so wide-eyed he'd stopped blinking. There was an unnerving stillness as the ground vibrated through their feet. It was as if they were at a rural train station with an express train due to hurtle through at any moment.

The remaining birds, until now hidden above, broke free of the trees and took to the sky as well, disappearing in a swirl of flapping wings, as the first two bikes burst into view.

The incomprehensible speed and ferocity in which they approached ripped at the group's faces like J. K. Rowling's Dementors. The long expanse of tarmac was eaten up in milliseconds, and, then, as quickly as the first wave of bikes had appeared, they were gone no sooner than they'd arrived.

Henk had seen it all before, and took great delight in watching the reactions of those experiencing it for the first time. He laughed loudly as he captured the gaping mouths of Frank and Stan on his camera.

"This is one crazy fuck-it-list event!" shouted Henk loudly.

Frank and Stan were dumbstruck, and barely had time to moisten their lips before the next volley of bikes arrived. The next two into view had been caught up on, so four bikes thundered through, inches from each other, ruffling the leaves on the trees as they passed in a blur. There was a kink in the road in front of them, and as every bike went by, the dip in the road caused the rider's heads to bob, like they were sharing a friendly exchange.

"Holy shit!" screamed Frank. "This is insane!"

It was overwhelming on the senses: the sight, the sound, and the smell. They didn't know whether to look at the bikes that'd just gone, or the ones just coming. Their heads spun back and forth like they were watching the fastest-ever game of tennis. It was exhilarating. For the next hour, the stream of bikes was constant.

The practice sessions were vital for less experienced riders to get a feel for the circuit and for seasoned professionals to reacquaint themselves. After all, this was an inhabited racetrack, and things like breaking points could have been painted, grown over, or simply moved since the previous year. It was also the time to take key readings on tyres, suspension set-up, anything that may eke out an extra mile an hour out of the bike. Qualifying lap times in practice week were also vital, because without enough completed laps at a qualifying speed, you were not permitted to race the following week.

With a number of classes to compete in on a number of different bikes, these guys weren't out for a gentle ride. The men and women risking everything for the challenge of racing the TT course was the culmination of months, and in many cases years, of work and determination. Frank and Stan weren't seasoned motorsport fanatics, but from the moment the first bike went by, they were hooked. It was nothing the likes of which they'd ever seen, or would do again — simply mesmerising.

With the sun falling in the sky, Frank assumed the evening's session was being brought to a close as the wonderful chaos in front of them eased to a deafening silence.

One of Henk's friends, Rudy — also a seasoned veteran aficionado, judging by his adornment of racing badges — grinned like a madman.

"Fooking amazing, no?" he said, gripping Frank and Stan around the shoulders.

The lads nodded in agreement, still somewhat stunned and ears ringing.

"Right! Sidecars next!" Rudy exclaimed, pulling a hip flask from his pocket, which he eagerly shared with his new friends.

Frank was almost embarrassed at the hospitality complete strangers were showing them, but the slug of smooth, expensive-tasting alcohol both eased his concerns and warmed his insides quite nicely now that the warming rays of the sun had disappeared behind the treeline.

The anticipation grew, once again, as the infectious enthusiasm of the radio commentator — Chris Kinley — radiated from the speakers, as he called away the sidecar competitors from the start line. There was barely chance to take a second nip from the hip flask before the sidecars broke the birds foolish enough to settle back into the trees from their reverie for a second time.

Frank thought about how he'd explain what he was seeing to his friends at home, but he couldn't. No matter how many videos, photographs, or detailed descriptions, it was simply unfathomable to anyone not fortunate enough to see it in person. The only way to truly appreciate it, properly appreciate it, was to actually be there. It now made perfect sense why people sat in a field all day, or hovered in a tree, to view the grand display.

They may not have been as quick as their solo counterparts, but the sidecars could shift, and unbelievably so. Stan and Frank marvelled as the 'chairs' hurtled past them, the riders once again bobbing their head as they negotiated the small dip in the road. They were every bit as impressive as those before, and it was difficult to conceive that two people were attached to these pieces of metal hurtling next to them.

Frank shook his head in dismay. "Dave and Monty must be absolutely bonkers to get on one of them things!" he shouted over the sound of the screaming engines.

The end of the sidecar session brought an end to Frank and Stan's TT debut. They were both emotionally drained, sporting a look of complete bewilderment. The smile on Frank's face dropped for a moment, as he said, "I can't believe I've waited so long to see that. We should have done this thirty years ago, Stan."

Stan smiled. "It's better than having never done it at all," he said. "Plus, we've got another two weeks of this to look forward to!"

Frank didn't respond. For a few moments, his brain was elsewhere.

"Hello, Frank, are you listening?" Stan asked.

Frank's attention was back, his brain now returned to his body. "We need to get a sidecar," he declared.

"I think we're a bit old for that, to be honest," said Stan. "Plus I'm not so sure I'd want to see you in tight leathers, no offence."

"Not for us, Stan," Frank replied with urgency and conviction. "We need to get a sidecar for Dave and Monty — well, at least an engine — I'm dead serious. There has got be somewhere on this island we can buy an engine. Stan, this is unbelievable. The racing, the Island, Henk, the boat, the... *everything.*"

Frank was a man possessed. Stan didn't dare interrupt him.

"I fucking love this place to pieces," Frank continued. "Just imagine how unbelievable it'd be to have a sidecar with our name on it. Well, the charity's, I mean," he said, now gripping Stan around the shoulders. "Stan, with the amount of money we have, we must be able to sort an engine out. We're not just going to be watching the races, my old friend. You and I are *going to be part of the races!*"

"I'm with you, mate," Stan said. "I love it to bits as well, only..."

"Only what?" Frank asked.

"Only, can you let go my shoulders?" Stan said. "Your bloody death-grip is hurting me, for fucksake!"

chapter twelve

nothing filled the bars and pubs of Liverpool more than a warm, balmy summer evening. The town centre was heaving as happy punters cast aside their suit jackets and ties, enjoying a drink or two after a day at the office. It was easy to forget the pain and fear of a bitter-cold winter's evening when drenched in the warming rays.

Arthur Hughes enjoyed the bustling crowds; it was easy for him to be anonymous and for a brief time, less vulnerable. It was difficult to retain a respectable appearance without washing facilities, but Arthur managed as best he could under the circumstances. His greying hair was a little more erratic than it once was, and the absence of a fresh razor blade meant the stubble on his face was irregular. He tried to dress as smartly as he could, if nothing else, for a fleeting feeling of normality. He'd aged more this past six months than the previous six years. His eyes were the biggest clue; the sparkling blue eyes of his youth were now hollow and sunken, and had virtually glossed over. He looked like a man who'd all but given up. And, in fact, this was precisely what he was.

"What are you staring at, you dirty git?" shouted a young city type clutching a large glass of red wine. "Are you simple or something? Stop looking at my girlfriend!" he added, much to the amusement of his colleagues.

Arthur shuffled uneasily; he tried to move away quickly but his loose-fitting slippers made it more difficult than it should have been.

"I'm... I'm sorry," he stuttered over his shoulders as he walked away.

"Pervert!" shouted the voice over the crowd. "Look at his bloody slippers!" it said, to an eruption of laughter.

"I thought she looked like someone," Arthur said quietly, "I'm sorry, she looked like someone I knew."

He continued to protest his innocence, mumbling to himself, long after they were out of earshot. A wave of emotion ran through him as he stood in a doorway and rubbed his ears furiously, like he was trying to start a fire. He sat on a concrete step and rubbed his eyes with the palms of his hands.

"I thought I knew her," he said aloud, to no one. "She looked familiar."

His coat was too big — ideal for winter, but stifling in this weather. He didn't live through the previous colder months; he existed. He couldn't afford to let go the coat, and if he tried to store it somewhere, he knew it'd be gone when he returned for it. His dark trousers were an inch or so too short for him, but fitted comfortably at the waist, which, like the compassion in his eyes, was slowly diminishing. His comfortable brown boots, which had served him well during the ice and snow, were, like everything he owned, taken from him. The peril of having something of use on the streets was that someone younger and stronger would take them at will. Arthur, even in his present condition, was no pushover, and those boots were vital for survival. He hadn't given them up without a fight, which was the reason for the savage-looking gash on his left cheek.

Lack of food was crippling, but what Arthur struggled with most was the lack of sleep. He couldn't remember the last time he slept more than two or three hours at a time. It helped not at all that, as soon as he found a place of relative safety, it was gone the following night and he was alone, once again, looking for a place to get his head down.

"Are you going to bed?" said a young voice.

Arthur took his head from his hands and looked quizzically at a young girl, no older than three or four, stood in front of him. She had a vibrant summer dress on and had her blonde hair tied up in bunches.

"Are you going to bed?" she asked, in reference to his slippers. "My mummy bought me some slippers, like yours, but mine don't have as many stains. Do you live in this house?" she continued at pace.

Arthur smiled and gently waved her away, but she stood and smiled. "Would you like a sherbet lemon?" she said, pulling a yellow sweet from her pocket. "I've got several. They're my favourite. Mummy doesn't know that I took them from the house."

"You should go," said Arthur gently.

"I'm Emily," she said, handing Arthur the yellow sweet.

"You shouldn't talk to strangers, Emily," said Arthur, taking the sweet in the hope it would usher her on her way.

She smiled and skipped up the road, humming a tune to herself. She stopped for a moment to unwrap the tightly-bound plastic wrapper separating her from her own lemon treat. She was oblivious to the speeding traffic in front of her, and continued to concentrate on the sweet that yet eluded her.

Arthur jumped up and shouted, "Emily!"

She didn't respond so Arthur quickened his pace. The slippers caused him to stumble, so he kicked them to one side.

"Emily!" he shouted, louder this time. He broke into a jog as he continued to call after her. "Stop there, sweetheart!"

She took a step onto the road and startled traffic swerved from the nearside lane to take avoiding action. The screeching tyres finally broke Emily's concentration, but her momentum took her a further pace into the road.

Arthur lunged forward and caught the collar of her dress, throwing her toward the pavement. A black taxi skimmed millimetres from Arthur, and the passenger-side wing mirror clipped him just above the waist. If Emily had still been in the road, the impact would have been directly on her head. The collision knocked Arthur off his feet and he landed awkwardly on top of Emily, who, by now, had naturally started to scream.

Barefoot and not as mobile as he once was, Arthur flailed on the pavement, unable to get to his feet. Several bystanders moved cautiously toward the pair, unsure what exactly was going on. Emily continued to scream, as a trickle of blood ran down her knee onto her white ankle socks.

Arthur managed to roll over onto his front, and pushed himself into praying position before using a black bin as leverage to get back to standing. He was in pain and had lacerations on his feet, but his first thought was for the little girl. She tried to smile at him, but the tears prevailed as she sobbed uncontrollably.

Several bystanders moved to assist, closely followed by a hysterical woman who took Emily in her arms.

"Baby, baby, I only turned my back for one moment," she said, caressing the girl's hair, and wiping her bloodied knee with a handkerchief.

"Baby, what happened?"

Emily took a laboured breath in between sobs, and pointed to Arthur. "That man," she said.

Her mother squeezed her as she looked askance at Arthur, a mixture of dismay and disgust on her face. Arthur knew he looked a state, which certainly didn't help her opinion of him.

One of the onlookers was a burly workman, and faced with the situation before him, took a firm grip on Arthur's arm and shoved him away from the girl.

"I pushed her," said Arthur. "I didn't mean to hurt her."

The workman was initially the aggressor, but as the baying mob — including Emily's mother — heard that Arthur had pushed her, became the calming influence as he placed a protective arm around Arthur, preventing a physical assault.

Arthur was pushed into the shop doorway from where the mother had appeared, but he had trouble maintaining coherency and could only mumble to himself incessantly.

"The old bastard's mental!" shouted one voice.

"Should be strung up!" shouted another.

Arthur's heart smashed in his chest as a cloud of angry faces floated in front of him.

"I've phoned the old bill!" shouted a store security officer, who moved to calm the situation. He took Arthur by the arm and guided him inside the shop, away from the angry mob. Once inside, Arthur took one final look back toward Emily. Her sobs had given way to a smile, and she held her palm to show him the yellow boiled sweet, finally undone, in her hand.

"I need my slippers," Arthur said to no one. "I can't go anywhere without my slippers."

Arthur sat alone and scared atop of a thin blue plastic mattress in a cold custody suite. Still, though he knew it was irrational, the thought of a safe, secure night's sleep was becoming appealing. The banging and screaming from the neighbouring cells, on the other hand, disturbed him greatly. Arthur pushed his knees into his chest and he buried his head, holding his ears to drain out the noise.

He didn't hear the cell door open.

"Arthur, come on mate, you're free to go," said a firm but gentle voice.

Arthur followed the young officer without question. He was brought to the same sergeant's desk where he'd been processed a few hours earlier.

"You're free to go, no charges," said the sergeant. "Do you need a lift anywhere?" he added, not unkindly.

The younger officer took Arthur to one side, and explained to him that the girl had told her mother what had happened and that they'd been into the station as soon as they were able.

"The young girl asked me to give you this," said the officer. "I think it's a lemon sherbet? She said not to worry as she's got another."

Arthur bowed his head and brushed his cheek, which had suddenly gone wet.

"I can go?" asked Arthur.

"Not quite yet, I'm afraid," said the officer. "By the way, my name is Darren. Wait there for a moment, please?"

Darren came back with a bag, from which he produced a pair of immaculate black walking boots. "Size seven? We could only guess, but the shop said you can change them no problem if you need to."

Arthur looked up at the officer, confused.

"Ah. Well, you see, when we found out what had happened, we went to look for your slippers. We found them, sure enough, but they were a mess. And so all the team on shift threw some money in to buy you some boots. I hope you don't mind? You know, about the slippers? Oh, and we've also got some clothes left from lost-property. all cleaned. Please, help yourself."

After a bit, the sergeant handed him a pile of leaflets on where the homeless could get help, such as accommodation and food. In truth, Arthur had exhausted all of the available options, but he was so grateful for a moment of compassion that he took them anyway, gratefully. His boots were a perfect fit and the clothes from lost property were deeply appreciated. He didn't keep his existing wardrobe apart from the coat, which kept him warm in winter.

"One more thing," said Darren. "There's someone who wants to talk with you at the front desk."

Darren escorted him and gave him a friendly pat on the back.

"Take care, okay?" the officer said fondly, then nodded at the man waiting patiently on a wooden bench in the reception area.

"Arthur?" asked the man politely.

Arthur looked back at the policeman, who gave him a reassuring nod, and then to the new fellow again. "Yes, I'm Arthur," he said cautiously.

"Great!" said the new fellow. "Arthur, my name is Lee Watson, and I work for a charity called Frank 'n' Stan's Food Stamps. It's not the catchiest, I know, but the clue is in the name. Can we grab a coffee?"

Arthur was suspicious. After months of living on the streets, it was difficult to be anything but, but he gratefully took a mug of hot tea and a large bacon bap and listened to Lee.

Lee had clearly indulged since his time on the streets, sporting a rather impressive paunch, but his enthusiasm was equally as impressive. He spoke with passion about his own time spent homeless, and his chance meeting with Frank and Stan. Arthur felt an empathy with Lee because he'd been in the very same situation Arthur currently found himself, albeit Lee being considerably younger.

"Arthur, in short, I'm part of a charity who gives food stamps out to the homeless. We're not the first and hopefully we won't be the last, but we want to ensure that the homeless are getting at least one hot meal a day. Here's a list where you can collect the vouchers, and here's a list where you can redeem them. They have no cash value so cannot be exchanged for alcohol or drugs. We know there are food banks, Salvation Army, and other charities, but they're struggling to cope. This way, you can be sure to get a healthy warm meal every day. Well until the money runs out, at least!"

Arthur frowned, but Lee did his best to reassure him.

"Arthur, honestly, there's no catch. Just a bunch of people hoping to do some good — that's it. We just want people to spread the word. The guys at the police station have been great, calling us when they have someone they think we can help, I hope you don't mind? Do you have any questions?"

Arthur took a mouthful of his tea and sat in silence for a moment. The tea was hot and he could feel himself warming. His vision blurred as his eyes welled up.

"Are you okay?" asked Lee, "can I do anything? If you need me to get you a lift somewhere, that's no problem? Arthur?"

Arthur dabbed at his eyes with a napkin, and, then, vision clear, took a look down at his new boots.

"I got these new boots," he said, admiring them. "I was happy for a brief moment, but then I realised that someone would see them and want to take them and I'd end up with another black eye. I was almost tempted to give them back and go barefooted — at least then people would leave me alone. But then I thought that, at least with these boots, I could walk further — or, in this case, climb further."

"Climb?" asked Lee, uncertainly.

"Yes, climb. The only positive thing I could think about these shoes, at least at first, was that I could walk in comfort to the highest building I could find." Arthur took a picture from his inside pocket and held it out. "Lee, I was going to take this picture of my daughter, climb a building, any would do, the taller the better, and jump from it."

The blood drained from Lee's face. "Mate. You're not going to, you know, jump in front of a train, or something stupid?" he asked.

"No, Lee, I'm not," Arthur continued. "That was my plan, but not anymore. I've seen more compassion today, in this one day, than I have taken altogether in a good long while. The thought of a warm meal each day, for me, is more than you can possibly imagine. Well, then again, I suppose you *can* and *have* imagined."

Arthur was beginning, tentatively, to feel human once again.

"Am I safe to leave you?" asked Lee.

"You're fine, Lee, I promise," said Arthur.

"Here's my phone number, Arthur," Lee said, extending to him a card. "If I can help, I will. Please don't hesitate to ask. I've got plans to extend the remit of the charity, so hopefully we can help more also, you know, with accommodation and that."

Lee stood, preparing to go, and gave Arthur the look of a concerned parent. "Arthur, I'm going to meet you tomorrow, and help you find somewhere to live," he said.

"I'm okay, Lee. You've done something special today, and, please, can you tell your friends Frank and Stan that as well."

Arthur took another sip of hot tea.

"Lee," Arthur said to Lee, now at the door. "Thank you for treating me with dignity."

Arthur sat, cuppa in hand, and smiled to himself. He looked at his boots once more, considering them. They really were quite nice, no complaints. And the clear moonlit sky predicted a welcome night on the street, free from the common wet British weather so often experienced. Arthur felt positive. He took a deep breath in, straightening his back, and raising his shoulders up.

Suddenly, Lee burst back through the door, shaking his head.

"I can't bloody leave you to sleep out there tonight!" exclaimed Lee. "Don't think I'm mad — well I am, just not weird or anything — but you can come home with me tonight, and we'll get you sorted with something. I'm not sure what, but we'll sort something out!"

"Right. Can I finish my tea first?" Arthur asked.

chapter thirteen

"this must be the street," said Stan, examining a crude map drawn on the back of an envelope. "What's the point in having a mobile phone if you don't answer it," he continued, more a statement then a question.

"Maybe he's sleeping," replied Frank. "It is only eight a.m., after all"

The two walked along an unassuming row of red-brick terraced houses, each with a small garden to the front.

Stan crumpled the paper in frustration. "Do they not know how to put numbers on the front of these bloody houses?"

Frank was a few paces in front, and peered over a small wall. "I'm going to take an educated guess that this is the one," he said.

Stan quickened his pace. "There's no number."

"Yes," said Frank. "But there's an empty beer can in the garden."

"Doesn't mean it's Dave's house?" Stan answered, nearly caught up.

"It does when it's still in Monty's hand," replied Frank.

"Ah," said Stan.

Monty lay motionless, his arms wrapped around a garden gnome in a manner which appeared very much one of great affection.

"I think he likes that gnome a bit too much," said Frank.

"No, it's okay," said Stan, now in the garden and leaning over Monty. "He's just got a mobile phone in his pocket, is all."

"Let's hope that's all it is," Frank replied.

"Wait, hang on," said Stan.

"Is he alive?" asked Frank.

"The gnome is broken," said Stan. "It's busted right down the middle."

"Correction, then," Frank offered. "I think he *liked* that gnome a bit too much... quite literally. Anyhow, I meant what state is Monty in?"

"Well I'm not a bloody doctor, am I," protested Stan.

"I know, but you understand the concept of air coming out of the nose or mouth as an indication that someone is alive? Hold your hand over his mouth."

Stan knelt down, giving Monty a good once-over. He took a hesitant 'why me?' glance at Frank, before slowly lowering his hands down to Monty's face.

"Anyways, it's too breezy," he said. "I can't hear if he's breathing."

"Put your ear to his mouth," suggested Frank.

Stan adjusted his position and lowered his head. Monty was a considerable unit, and Stan struggled to get in a comfortable position to listen to him breathing. He had to place a hand either side of Monty's chest as he listened intently.

"Well?" asked Frank. "Can you hear him breathing?"

"No, but he's definitely alive," called back.

"How can you tell?" Frank said, confused.

"I can smell his breath, and trust me, it's not good. *He's* alive, but it smells like something has gone and died in his *mouth.* You're going to have to help me up, now, as I'm feeling a bit faint."

Frank stood over the two of them, unsure of how best to approach this. He intended to crouch down, put his hands under Stan's armpits and help him up... but as he moved forward, Monty roused briefly from his slumber. His face contorted with fear and panic when he saw Frank stood above him and Stan crouched beside him. Most disconcerting, at least to Frank, was that, through the benefit of his lazy eye, Monty was able to focus one eye on each of them — independently.

Monty made a garbled scream and instinctively kicked out to protect himself. His right foot rose majestically, and the toe of his heavy boot caught Frank squarely in the bollocks.

The air flew out of Frank's lungs as a wave of agony ascended through his body like a lightning bolt. He wailed in pain, cupping his throbbing testicles. His legs, now like jelly, gave out, and he dropped to his knees, leant over, his head come to rest a few mere inches south of Monty's groin. Monty's incoherent mumbling was drowned out by Frank praying to a higher power to relieve the agony he was in.

Without the offered assistance, Stan was unable to right himself. This left them, currently, a tangle of limbs — with Monty still clutching the garden gnome under one arm, Frank in pain and virtually in tears next to Monty's crotch, and Stan at Monty's throat, with grunting noises from the exertion, trying desperately to... well, it wasn't quite clear *what* he was trying to do at this point.

"Help me!" screamed Monty, becoming lucid. "I'm being violated!"

Mrs Timpson — Dave's long-suffering neighbour — was on her morning rounds with her chihuahua, Frodo. Alerted by the various screams, she picked up her dog, placing a protective arm around it. "I'll phone the police!" she warned, as she looked apprehensively into the garden.

She stood with her mouth agape and instinctively covered Frodo's eyes to protect him from the imagined depravity that was on display before her. There sat Monty, laid on his back, Stan making *Unh-unh-unh!* noises at his neck, and Frank making *Ah-ah-ah!* noises at his crotch. And, in the middle of all this, was an abused garden gnome.

"You disgust me, you, you... bloody deviants!" she shouted, retreating up the street. "Come on, Frodo!" she added, though Frodo could do nought else, being as he was still in Mrs Timpson's arms.

"It's not what it looks like!" Frank, who'd managed to get some air back into his lungs, called after her. "It's only a mobile phone he's got in his pocket!" he insisted, grabbing the bulge in Monty's pocket to emphasise the point.

Frank struggled to his feet and used the last of his energy to pull Stan upright.

"We're going to get bloody arrested," said Stan. "And how the hell has he fallen back to sleep?" he added, looking at Monty, who was curled up, once again, with his garden gnome.

"I don't know," said Frank. "But I feel compelled to tell you... that was *not*, in fact, a mobile phone in his pocket."

Frank rattled the knocker — shaped like a sidecar — on the white, plastic door, but no answer was immediately forthcoming.

Stan looked nervously up the street. "We need to get the hell out of here," he said. "Being arrested for violating Monty and a garden ornament is not how I want to be remembered."

"The ornament was like that when we arrived," Frank assured him. "Wait there," he said, wincing in pain, his bollocks still hurting, and he jockeyed around for a better view inside.

"I think I can see movement," he announced after a few productive minutes of peeping.

Frank rattled the door several times further before a shadow became apparent, looming through the frosted glass.

The door opened, and Dave filled the frame. Like the first time they met, Dave was once again sporting a pair of oil-stained Y-fronts, only this time, regrettably, there was no t-shirt to spare his modesty — just a pair of underpants and a generous stomach, an image that was starting to burn an unholy imprint on Frank's retinas, but was nevertheless a welcome distraction from his pain.

"You pair been mucking about, having fun with Monty?" asked Dave cheerily.

"Dave," said Frank slowly. "You do know that you've got a toothbrush in your hair and what looks like the remains of a chocolate digestive stuck to your right... breast."

Dave rubbed his eyes, yawned, and looked down onto his chest. "McVitie's. They're the best, aren't they? I seem to recall I was looking for that last night, after it'd gone missing. Cheers."

"Look, Dave. Henk took us out to watch the practices last night..." Frank started to say, but the big man was only half-listening.

Dave plucked what was left of the McVitie's chocolate digestive from the tangle of his chest hairs and popped it into his mouth. The toothbrush, he did not remove; he left it right where it was, and, grasping the handle, used it to scratch his head. He munched on the digestive contentedly.

"It's pretty special," Dave said thoughtfully, though it was unclear if he was referring to the TT practices or the biscuit. "So, anyway, what's up?"

"Henk took us out to watch the practices last night," Frank explained again. "And, well, it's the most remarkable thing we've ever seen. I can understand how this thing gets into your blood, into your soul."

"Mm-hmm," Dave agreed.

"Anyway," continued Frank. "I know you've met Henk before. But did you know that he's got loads and loads of motorsport memorabilia in his house? You know, ones that he's sponsored over the years?"

"I didn't, but go on," said Dave, who'd now pulled the toothbrush from his hair, inspected it, and, apparently satisfied it still had remnants of toothpaste on it, set about giving his teeth a bit of a spot clean.

"Well, he's got a sidecar at the bottom of his stairs, and it's only the twenty-fourteen world championship-winning sidecar," Frank said.

"Twenty-thirteen, I think," interrupted Stan.

"Whatever year it is, it won a world championship," continued Frank. "Apparently, Henk was the main sponsor. And, guess what!"

Dave's eyes widened. "He's going to let me use the engine?"

Frank looked a bit deflated. "No, but to be honest, we did ask him. But he started to laugh."

"And I think he was still laughing when we left the house, in fact," added Stan, interrupting once again.

"So why did you word it like that?" asked Dave. "Like you were coming to the door with the offer of a world-championship-winning sidecar engine? You can see why I'd think that, don't you?"

"You're right, Dave. And, sorry, I didn't mean to get your hopes up too much. I just meant to set the scene, you know, about Henk being into sidecars in a big way," explained Frank.

"So, can Henk get me an engine?" asked Dave, his hopes once again piqued.

"Well, no," Frank said.

"So you've woken me and Monty up to tell me that you saw a nice sidecar?" Dave said, getting visibly irritated.

Stan didn't say a word. He simply let Frank carry on, seeing as how he was doing so well at it.

"Well, yes, but I can get you an engine," Frank said. "Just not from Henk, from one of his friends that's staying with him," he elaborated.

Dave was tired and confused, so Frank clarified further.

"Right, it's like this, Dave. One of Henk's friends also sponsors a few of the bike riders, and he's offered to sell us a Suzuki 600, whatever the technical name you called it, that you can put in your sidecar. It's raced before and it's good to

130

go, apparently. There's just this one thing — it's one of the spare engines the McMullan brother was going to use."

"You're joking?" asked Dave.

"No, it's not cheap. But don't worry about that, After we watched the practices, we wanted to be involved, didn't we, Stan?"

Stan nodded. "We did," he agreed, now that it was somewhat safe to speak. "But one thing, Dave. Don't take this the wrong way, but Henk's friend would only sell it if you guys were serious about racing."

"We're serious," said Dave immediately "Dead serious. Serious as the grave."

"I know," continued Stan. "We know that well enough. But, see, this fella, he was almost coming with us this morning, and he'd have been greeted by..."

Stan swept his hand in front of him expansively, like a game show host's lovely assistant highlighting a prospective prize on display just revealed to the audience.

"Greeted by what?" asked Dave, getting more frustrated.

"Well," said Stan, coughing uncomfortably. "You've got your passenger asleep in your garden, for instance, and he looks like he's spent the entire night making love to Papa Smurf, and—"

"We love who we love," Dave interrupted.

"And you're walking around in your underpants," Stan continued. "With a hangover, and with a biscuit stuck to your chest."

"What? Did I miss some?" Dave asked, examining his chest to see if there were perhaps more breakfast available.

Dave looked as if he was going to say something else, possibly in his defence, when Stan took a step forward and looked past him into the sitting room.

"Dave, hang on," Stan said. "But is that a bloke asleep, standing up, or have you nailed him to the wall?"

Dave turned and started to chuckle. "Ah, that's James," he said, as if this should be enough of an explanation in itself. Seeing that it was not, he continued, "The sofa must have been taken, and he's pretty good a sleeping upright. You know. Like a cow or a horse — whichever one of those sleeps standing up, I can't remember. I'm not so good with farm animals."

"That would surprise me," Stan said.

Dave faced Stan, with a solemn look on his face. "We're serious about racing," he said. "The only reason we're like this today is because we were so devastated about not being able to race. Monty was in tears all night, and I've started to comfort eat, once again," he said, pointing to the ring of chocolate on his chest left where the McVitie's had been. "We've lived this for the last twelve months, and the bottom of our world dropped out when the reality that it was all for nothing sunk in."

Stan held his hands up. "No offence meant, Dave. I was just worried that if he'd seen you this morning, he may have changed his mind, that's all."

"He doesn't know you like we know you, is all," Frank added.

"So... we've got an engine?" Dave ventured.

Frank smiled. "Yes, we do indeed have an engine."

"Why didn't you just say so at the start!" shouted Dave excitedly.

"He had to, y'know, set the scene," said Stan.

James, stirred by Dave's shouting, snorted once, clomped his foot to the floor several times, then settled back to sleep, still standing up.

"I've got the guy's number," Frank went on. "He said if you call him, you can meet him, and it's pretty much ready to go. You should be able to go out tonight, in fact. That is, if you two have sobered up enough?"

James whinnied. He was dreaming.

"We'll be fine, I can promise you that!" insisted Dave. "And I cannot wait to see the look on that bell-end Harry McMullan's face when he knows I've got one of his engines!"

"Probably best if we didn't mention that, actually," suggested Stan diplomatically. "He's no fan of McMullan either, but the guy didn't want to cause any trouble around the paddock."

"Hmph. Well I suppose I see your point," Dave said, licking his finger and rubbing it round the crown of chocolate on his chest so he could enjoy every last bit.

"Oh, and we've been on the phone," Stan added. "And your pitch at the grandstand is still available!"

Dave began to perform his finest truffle-shuffle, and for a gentleman with a larger figure he could move surprisingly smoothly and rhythmically. Mesmerised, Stan had to shake his head to break the spell, as the motion of Dave's breasts jiggling — with the one glistening — was almost hypnotic.

"We're going racing, Monty! We're only going racing!" Dave repeated over and over, calling outside to the garden in celebration as he danced.

Monty didn't stir, so Dave went out to him, moved the gnome unceremoniously to one side, jumped on top of him, and, finding purchase, began dry-humping his leg.

"We're going racing!" Dave shouted, and between the shouting and the humping, Monty was finally roused.

"Bloody perverts!" shouted Mrs Timpson again, returning from her morning walk just in time to witness still more debauchery. "Don't look, Frodo," she insisted, though she already had Frodo's eyes well covered.

Dave gripped Monty by the ears, holding them out, the better with which to capture the sound of his shouting. "We've got an engine, Monty, we've got a bloody engine!"

Monty opened one eye — his good one — and clenched his fist in delight. "You little beauty!" he shouted. "You're being serious? You're not having me on?"

"That I am, Monty. That I am. We're packing up the van, heading back to the grandstand, and, tonight, Monty my old son, you're going to squeeze your tight little arse into your racing leathers."

Dave jumped around the garden, dancing, and generally scaring those heading off to their work, frightening the children, and spooking the horses.

There was a whinny, came from inside the house.

"Monty, and just one more thing," Dave called out.

"Wut's that?" Monty asked. "You mean there's more?"

"Naw, it's just, you really need this," Dave said, handing him his toothbrush. "No offence, mate. But you could strip paint with that breath."

Monty took the toothbrush, inspected it, and, apparently satisfied it still had remnants of toothpaste on it, set about giving his teeth a bit of a spot clean.

chapter fourteen

tuesday evening practice session.
    Stan paced back and forth.
    "I feel sick. Honestly, I could throw up," he said, rubbing his stomach for maximum effect.

"Have one of these," suggested Frank, handing him a cheeseburger. "This'll settle the nerves!"

"Has Dave been back in touch?" asked Stan, checking his phone again. "Do you think the engine was overpriced?"

Frank checked his phone as well. "Nothing since the last call, and no, I don't think we paid too much. The only thing overpriced is this bloody burger," said Frank, now grimacing at the plastic cheese dripping onto the saturated grease-proof paper.

"The money is all relative anyhow," Frank continued on. "We have it, and look what we've been able to do. We've got Dave and Monty back in the TT races, we'll get good advertising for the charity, and when was the last time you were this excited. Tell me you've ever been this brought to life by having money just sat in your bank account?"

The novice, but eager, team sponsors were stood at the foot of Bray Hill, one of the most iconic spots on the entire course — a steep, downhill section of the course which, when negotiating, must have felt like riding off the edge of the earth. Unsure of their directions, Frank and Stan had arrived early, before the roads closed, and watched the locals commute before the start of the practice session.

It was difficult to conceive that bikes would soon be hurtling down the hill at speeds of up to 170 mph inches from where they stood. It was still early in practice week, but the crowds began to descend on the popular vantage point.

"Chuck me one of those beers, will you?" asked Stan, "That will drown out the butterflies."

"Ooh, phones ringing," said Frank. "Hello."

Frank listened for a moment before shaking his head and covering the mouthpiece. "It's Stella, not Dave," he said before listening again. "Okay, okay, okay, Stella, you don't need to shout at me."

"She's upset about something!" whispered Frank to Stan, the phone held away at arm's length, ensuring Stella was out of range.

"Why? What's she on about?" Stan asked.

Frank shrugged his shoulders and prepared for a second salvo. He placed the phone back against his ear.

"Stella, take the fag out of your mouth and take a deep breath — of air, luv, not the fag. What's up?"

Those spectators near to Frank eased a little closer, hoping, no doubt, to eavesdrop on this juicy convo that must have sounded to them, from what they could hear, very much like an outraged wife chastising her husband for venturing out to the races.

Frank paid the interlopers no mind and listened intently, periodically moving the phone away from his ear to protect his tympanic membrane. Confused, he leaned toward Stan and asked, "Who the hell is Arthur?"

It was Stan's turn to shrug his shoulders. "No idea, why?"

"She's going mad about someone called Arthur," Frank said. And, then, back into the phone, "Stella, calling your employers a couple of imbeciles is not very nice, not to mention poor business practice. We have no idea who this Arthur is."

"Oh. So Lee's employed him, has he?" said Frank. "Right. This is all news to..." He paused for a moment, listening, and then, "Ah. Oh, yes. *That* Arthur. Yes, we knew all about it and we told him you'd give him a warm welcome, which, from what you've just said, sounds like you've given him."

Stan laughed silently, his shoulders bobbing up and down.

"Anyway, Stella, it sounds like you've got everything in hand over there," Frank told her. "I must go because we're having a can of something cold, presently, before the practices start. Okay... okay... yes... yes, lovely to speak with you as well. Cheers."

"What did she say?" asked Stan.

"She told me to stick my can of beer up your arse... and then drink it."

Stan nodded his head. "Nice. Yes, that's certainly our Stella, bless her. Anyway, so who's this Arthur fella?"

"No idea. I didn't want Stella to think we didn't know — it's not good for staff discipline. She's a bit upset because some 'mumbling old codger' has joined Lee working in the office. Apparently, he's helping Lee out with the charity. I'll give him a ring in a bit to see what's going on."

"Do you think we've made a good choice with Lee?" asked Stan.

"Well, the other reason she's upset is because she's been counting coins all day. Lee asked the drivers if they'd help out with a bit of fundraising and put a collection in their cars. In two days, they've raised just over three thousand pounds."

"That's amazing," said Stan.

"It's bloody brilliant! Stella said the safe in the office is almost bursting."

Once again, the sidecars were due to go out on the later session, after the solo bikes. Stan and Frank didn't have Henk or his radio with them tonight, but a giant speaker near where they stood blared out Radio TT for the benefit of those assembled. The viewing numbers had swelled considerably by this point, and unlike their location the previous evening, they were not covered by trees, and they basked in the gloriously sunny Manx evening. The atmosphere was electric and the anticipation in the air was palpable, and the commentator on the radio was getting more excitable as the start of the session approached.

Fortunately, due to their early arrival, they had a prime viewing spot, with a crowd approximately ten or eleven deep behind them. Parents stood with eager children wearing ear protectors on their shoulders. The still calmness of the empty road was, once again, unnerving and slightly eerie — but it only enhanced the feeling of anticipation.

As soon as the commentator called the first two riders away, the crowd stood to attention and stretched their necks out. The start line was out of view — only half-a-mile or so up the road — and the noise of the engines echoed through the still air.

The arrival of the first two bikes a moment later was an outright assault on the senses, and, from seeing sedate traffic a short while earlier, to bikes hurtling past them now, was epic. They were stood near a traffic light with a protective cushion wrapped around it, but, with the speed the participants were going, a bouncy castle between them wouldn't have been much use if the riders didn't navigate the gentle right-hander at the foot of the hill.

There was a slight dip in the road, which wasn't apparent to the naked eye, and Frank nearly ended up on top of Stan when the first rider bottomed out his machine — causing a stream of brilliant sparks to fly out from the bottom of the fairing — before disappearing up Quarterbridge Road.

"Holy shit!" screamed Stan. "That's unbelievable!"

Stan wasn't the only one grinning like a schoolboy. Everyone around them had the same reaction. There was even a schoolboy next to them — sat on his dad's shoulders —

grinning like a schoolboy, and doing an especially good job of it.

"I've been going to the football for years," Frank told Stan during a brief recess in the action. "And this beats football no end!"

They, like most of the crowd, stood slack-jawed for the remainder of the solo session, which went on for over an hour. The action was breathtaking.

There was a brief lull after the last of the solos roared by.

"My ears are ringing," said Frank. "Sidecars next!"

"Give me another beer, will you?" asked Stan, "My stomach's flipping something crazy."

It was getting later in the evening, and the crowd had thinned out slightly. Stan was pacing back and forth once more. "Our friend's in this," he was saying, to himself as much as to anyone willing to listen. "He's got one of the fastest engines out there!" he added, like he knew what he was talking about.

The screaming of an engine over the loudspeaker signalled the departure of the first sidecar. The sidecars were set off on their own, ten seconds apart, and it wouldn't be long at all before the first of them made its appearance.

"What number are they again?" shouted Stan.

Frank raised his fingers and signalled a four and a two.

"Our friend's forty-two!" announced Stan, like an expectant father, to those within earshot. "We're his sponsors!" he explained, to make clear that he and Frank were the proud parents.

Frank counted the sidecars down till they were approaching forty.

"Any minute now," said Frank. "Get your camera ready!"

Thirty-nine, forty, forty-one, and then forty-three and forty-four passed by...

"What happened? Did I miss them?" asked Stan, popping his head up from behind his camera phone.

"I don't think so?" Frank offered.

Eventually, Number Forty-Two trundled past, visibly slower than any of the other bikes had been.

"He wasn't exactly flying, was he?" Stan said.

Frank shook his head. "No, it didn't look like it. Did you manage to get a photo, then?"

"Get a photo? He was going that slow I could have painted a watercolour of him! Still, at least everyone could get a good look at the charity logo. It did look quite nice. Maybe that's his game?" wondered Stan.

"Or maybe he's just getting used to the track again?" suggested Frank.

"He's cagey," offered Stan. "Playing it close to the vest. It looked like he sped up a bit after he went by, though?"

"Stan, can you get that app working on your phone? The timing one Henk told us about?" Frank asked.

The two watched the live timing feed, which showed the competitors as they passed through timing beacons located at key points around the course.

"There he is!" shouted Stan. "He's still going."

Frank put his arm around Stan as they stood in the middle of a patch of grass, next to dozens of people they'd never met, listening to a giant speaker, and sharing a look at Stan's mobile phone. It was surreal, but also strangely compelling.

"Go on, Dave and Monty!" shouted Stan. "We sponsor them," he said, looking around, proper chuffed, in case people had missed it the first time.

"It looks like they've found their rhythm, they've started to pick up the pace, "he said to Frank. "Go on, you beauties!" he bellowed at the phone.

They were gripped as Dave broke the timing beacon at both the Glen Helen section and the famous Ballaugh Bridge — where bikes would often become airborne, making for a spectacular photo opportunity.

The radio commentary enhanced the experience, and Frank and Stan erupted as the announcer gave a mention to Team Frank 'n' Stan, and how Dave was a late entry and nearly didn't make it.

"That's us!" shouted Stan, giving a high-five to those within reaching distance.

Those around them didn't turn their nose up at these two excitable idiots; they shared in their joy, and because they were part of all this, they seemed to understand their excitement perfectly well.

The riders first out were soon approaching the grandstand at the end of their lap, and the air growled in the distance with the sound of raw horsepower. The backmarkers, which included Dave and Monty, were yet to break the beam at the Ramsey Hairpin — a challenging part of the track located near to the twenty-fifth milestone.

Frank hit the refresh button on the phone.

"Should he not be there by now? Number Fifty-Two is showing ahead of them."

They waited, impatiently, desperate for an update. By now, those stood near them were caught up in the enthusiasm, arching their necks to follow progress of Dave and Monty.

Frank looked at Stan. "Where the hell is...?"

One of the marshals stood a few feet from their location moved at pace, and began frantically waving a red flag.

"What's he doing? What's going on?" Said Frank, looking at those around him for an answer.

Outfit Number Three, which had begun their second lap, eased gracefully to a stop in front of them.

"Why's he stopped?" continued Frank.

The man with the child on his shoulder took a step back. "The race has been stopped," he explained.

"The race has been stopped," repeated the boy on the man's shoulders, in case Dad hadn't explained it well enough.

"Stopped? But why?" asked Stan. "Why would they stop it?"

Both Frank and Stan suspected they knew the answer, even though they were reluctant to hear it.

"It could be a number of reasons," the dad said sympathetically. "But, one of them is that there could have been an incident on the track."

Stan looked at Frank and then back to the man. "But it could be something else, yes?"

"Well, yes," said Dad.

"It could be something else," agreed Boy.

"If, for example, an ambulance had to get to a resident inside the course," offered the man. "Or an animal was loose. They would stop the race."

"If an animal was loose," added the boy helpfully.

The group moved closer to the radio loudspeaker, desperate for an update.

"They didn't make it to the next beacon. What if something's happened to them? What if we've given them an engine and something's happened to them," Frank said, the last more a statement than a question, with Frank contemplating the very real possibility.

Frank's mouth was dry. He looked for consolation from the faces around him, but it was not forthcoming. The jovial atmosphere was turned sombre the second the red flag had been waved. He took another look at his phone, willing Number Forty-Two to have appeared at Ramsey Hairpin, but it hadn't, and it was evident from the number of bikes that had overtaken them that Dave and Monty were missing.

"They must have broken down," said Stan, with little conviction. "Maybe a problem with the new engine?"

He was trying to convince himself as much as Frank, and Frank nodded his head, but he wasn't listening — his attention was focussed completely on the radio commentary for an update. But without a practice session to comment on, music was being played over the speakers in the interim. Unfortunately, this only served to heighten Frank and Stan's apprehension and frustration.

They stood in contemplation for what seemed like an absolute age. They'd only known Dave and Monty for a short while, but they were all of them a team now, and the wait was agony.

The music ended...

The sound of someone clearing his throat...

We've had news from Race Control.

This was Tim Glover, the announcer, of Radio TT.

There was a collective hush as the crowd hung on every word.

The announcer cleared his throat once again, before continuing...

I regret to report that there has been an incident near to the Sulby Straight section of the course. We have no information on those involved, but we've been told that the evening practice session will now be brought to a close. We'll update you as soon as we are given more information.

"Where's Sulby Straight?" said Frank, looking at the man with the child once again.

The man looked pale, and he took his son from his shoulders and placed him on the ground.

"Is it before Ramsey Hairpin?" Stan asked.

The father stood there, eyes raised up, working it out.

"I'm afraid it is," Dad said softly after a moment, his eyes returning down to earth. "If your friends went through Ballaugh Bridge, and didn't arrive at Ramsey Hairpin, then it is possible that they were in that section, near to the Sulby Straight."

"Near to the Sulby Straight," Boy said, his young face creased with genuine concern.

Frank put his hand to his head. He walked in a circle, feeling lost. He stared blankly at the red flag still being brandished by the marshal.

"Bloody hell, Stan, this doesn't look good." He took a deep breath and rubbed his forehead. "What if something has happened to Dave and Monty?"

"I don't know, mate," said Stan, the worry lines in his face showing prominently. "I don't know..."

chapter fifteen

Wednesday – Practice Week.
Arthur struggled with the chain coiled between two metal door handles. A rusty padlock gave the impression that the door was fastened securely, but — a spot of luck — a tug opened it up, with a bit of iron oxide dust falling to the floor.

"Let me," said Lee, pulling the heavy chain free.

"I'm thinking of taking up a self-defence class, Lee."

"Impressive," replied Lee, nodding his head in approval. "But you're not on the streets anymore. Is it more for fitness, then?"

"No, I'm starting to think I need to defend myself against that woman in the taxi office, Stella. She's a bit, ah... intimidating. She looks like she wants to attack me. Or eat me. I'm not sure which."

"She's a big lump, but she wouldn't attack you, Arthur!"

"I'm not so sure. I don't think she wants either of us in the office. She hid my chair today."

Lee patted Arthur on the back. "She's probably just teasing — you know, like some sort of taxi-related initiation."

"I don't know," said Arthur. "She spat in my cup of tea yesterday. Would that be considered a normal part of taxi-related initiations?"

"What??" Lee responded. "She wouldn't have done something like that, surely? How do you know?"

"I was holding the cup when she did it!" replied Arthur.

"We'll stick together, Arthur. Besides, we're only in there until Frank and Stan come back. They said we'll look for something elsewhere, so it's only a temporary measure."

Lee flicked the switch on his pocket torch, illuminating the dark brick walls which glistened from the light of the torch off fresh rainwater running down having taken advantage of the missing roof tiles. "You sure they're staying here? There doesn't seem to be much sign of life."

"I think so. Shine your torch over there, to the left of the chimney stack."

"What is this place?" asked Lee.

"I think it was a glazing factory, back in the day."

It was a vast expanse, but despite it being relatively warm outside, it was cold in the abandoned factory, with a damp chill in the air. The concrete floor was sodden with sporadic puddles of stagnant water. A row of inadequate windows spanned the upper third of the brick walls, but they'd long since succumbed to the elements — or possibly bored children using them for target practice.

"Ah, over there," said Lee.

There were piles of wooden pallets laid out on the floor, stacked just high enough that the makeshift covering gave the pile of blankets laid on top of them sufficient distance from the cold, wet floor.

Lee cautiously approached, holding the torch to the side of his head. "I don't think anyone's here, Arthur. Do you know how many stay here?"

Arthur shook his head. "No, I only stayed in here for a few nights... maybe eight or nine people? I think people moved on as quickly as they could. It's this dark and miserable in the middle of summer, so you can imagine what it was like in the middle of January. It was mostly younger people that stayed here, but there were an old couple as well, I don't know how old. They'd been married for years, I forget their names now."

"How'd they end up in this dump?" asked Lee.

"I think life just got the better of them both. They were injured in a car accident, couldn't work, and I imagine the bills stacked up, and they ended up here, in this. It's horrendous how life can turn on you."

Arthur looked like a different man after a few nights in a comfortable bed and a decent meal. With a proper shave and a haircut, he looked twenty years younger. The most apparent improved was that of his posture: he'd grown by at least two inches now he was no longer stooped over like a broken man.

"What about you, Arthur? I never asked how you ended up on the street," Lee said. "Tell me it's none of my business if you don't want to talk about it."

Arthur paused for a moment, after which were the sound of clinking glasses from where he'd tapped a pile of empty bottles strewn on the floor with the toe of his shoe.

"My biggest mistake, Lee, was that stuff — the demon drink. I was an alcoholic."

"I didn't think you drank?"

"I lost my wife to cancer. Fortunately, it was quick. But she went through a lot of pain. I'd only drank socially before that, but I think I started hitting it to numb the pain after she was gone."

"I'm sorry to hear that," Lee said sympathetically.

"My biggest regret is how I treated my daughter," Arthur continued. "When she needed me the most, I was drinking myself to death. I lost my business, the house, and everything I cared about. It was only when I'd lost everything that I stopped drinking. After I ended up on the street, I couldn't see the point even in drinking. I couldn't see the point in anything."

"What about your daughter?"

Arthur's eyes welled up. "She moved house and got married. I was so caught up with drinking, I didn't even walk my only daughter down the aisle. I'll never forgive myself for that. Never."

"I understand," said Lee.

"What about you, Lee?"

"My fate was all my own doing, Arthur. I did things I'm not proud off, got involved with some pretty despicable people — and I was one of them. I had to leave home pretty quickly, and, arriving in Liverpool with no money and a criminal record, there was only one place I was going to end up. Life is peculiar, though," Lee said. "Who'd have thought we'd meet up and be here, now, trying to help people out?"

"Life's a funny old thing," Arthur agreed.

"That it is," Lee replied. "Everything works out for a reason, I expect."

"There's nobody here," said Arthur, taking a final look into the pile of sheets. "We can leave a note letting them know where to come and get their food vouchers, yeah? Right, I should like to get out of here now. It really is bringing me back to an awful time in my life."

"Sure," said Lee, placing several flyers for the charity on the wooden pallets. "I'll be pretty glad to get out of this place myself," he agreed. "I think we've only got three or more buildings to do, and that's us handed out over one-hundred flyers, my old friend! That's pretty good going."

Lee put the lock and chain back as they'd found it, securing the door as best they could. There wasn't much to protect inside, but for the people who called this home it was all they had. He shuddered as they moved from the squalor, back into the warm, bright morning. "I wonder if the people in those posh apartments," he said, pointing up the street. "Just there. I wonder if they realise the conditions the homeless live in, only thirty seconds away from them?"

"I'm not sure most think about it," said Arthur. "Certainly, from my experience, most people try to ignore it, while some think that people *choose* that existence, even."

"No one would choose to live like that," agreed Lee. "Choosing to live like that would be completely mental. I mean, sure, there are some real scumbags living on the street. But there are some real scumbags anywhere you look. And most of the people I've met on the streets were honest, decent people, who'd just had a run of bad luck. Once you're down to nothing, it's exceptionally difficult to drag yourself back out again."

Lee paused for a moment, giving his phone a look.

"Shit, no way, Arthur!" he said. "That's Helen from the homeless shelter. She said they've had thirteen people in to collect food vouchers today, and these were people she'd never seen before. We've only been doing this for a few days. I'm well chuffed with that."

The positive news put a spring in both their steps, and spurred them on their mission to visit every derelict building in the city. It struck them that the official number of homeless could very well be significantly higher than reported. If they'd found thirteen people who'd never been to the shelter before, after all, how many more were there out there? How many more might there possibly be?

Arthur struggled to keep up with Lee, and chased him up the street like an excited puppy.

"You mean what you said, didn't you?" Arthur asked, finally at Lee's heels. "You know, about that woman in the taxi office?"

"About her not having a go at you? Of course I did," Lee said, stopping and allowing Arthur to catch up with him "Still. If she comes at us, fists swinging, me old chum, you're on your own I'm afraid. I want no part of that, as she'd give Mike Tyson a good workout!"

"Ta, that's very encouraging," Arthur said, and they both laughed as they carried on their mission.

chapter sixteen

frank's eyes were heavy from the gentle rocking of the carriage. His head bowed toward his chest before the shrill whistle from the engine brought him back to his senses.

"Stan, your sword. It keeps knocking me on the shin."

"Sorry!" replied Stan, his attention fixed outside the window. "This is amazing, you know — the countryside, and the smell. Everything. Look at this carriage," he said, though still looking out the window. It must be a hundred years old."

The sound of the train was amplified when they passed through a tunnel. They were briefly thrown into darkness and with nowhere for the steam to escape, the nostalgic aroma of a bygone time filled the carriage. Once through the tunnel, the fresh light abruptly revealed new scenery outside, as well as illuminating a small tableau inside the carriage — a young boy with his grandparents, sat with his nose pressed against the window, watching the rolling Manx hills pass before his eyes.

"Stan, it's hitting me again. Did you really need to buy a plastic sword?"

"It's for my neighbour's boy. He'll love this," said Stan, swinging it for effect like he was on the battlefield.

"So why did you buy yourself a helmet and a shield?" asked Frank. "And why are you wearing it now?"

"You can't go into battle without a shield and a sword to protect you. Isn't that right, young man?" Stan said conspiratorially to the young boy with his nose pressed to the window. They'd seen him earlier, walking around Castle Rushen, and he'd clearly persuaded his grandparents to be generous in the gift shop as he was now dressed impressively like a knight.

The boy seemed grateful for the attention, and raised his sword, grinning. He looked at Grandparents for the required approval before launching a playful assault on Stan, who used his shield to deftly repel the attack. The grandparents smiled indulgently, though appeared wary of the strange man sat opposite, across the aisle, engaged in battle. Ultimately, they must have regarded him as harmless — or perhaps somewhat mentally deficient, poor chap — as they allowed the campaign to rally on.

Frank was grateful for a relaxing day on the tourist trail. The last few days had been hectic, and the stress of the red flag the previous evening had played heavily on his mind. Fortunately for all concerned it had been only an oil leak — a fairly extensive one, but nothing more serious than that, thank goodness. The time it would take to clean up the track had meant the practice session was cancelled for the evening, was all.

As the train meandered from Castletown toward Douglas, Frank was once again transported back to his childhood, riding a train very much like the one they were in. In fact, it may well have been the very same train. He chuckled as he could almost hear his parents scolding him for putting his head too close to the open window. He looked at the young boy sharing their journey, so full of energy and enthusiasm, and wondered if the child, like he, would one day fondly relive the experience. Frank could vividly recall the wonderment at walking around Castle Rushen as a child. That in itself was a memorable experience, but, to travel there and back on steam train, for a child, was a wonderful adventure all unto itself.

"Are you okay over there?" asked Stan. "You seem unusually quiet." Stan had finally put down his sword. From the smile on the boy's face, it was obvious who'd won the battle.

"Fine, Stan, thanks. Just thinking. And remembering."

Stan gave him a knowing smile before returning attention to his former opponent, who was now issuing Stan the terms of surrender.

The railway heritage on the Island was magical, and for enthusiasts — similar to the TT devotees — it was easy to understand why a visit to this wonderful island was a privilege.

"My clothes smell of the train," said Stan, sniffing himself, walking up the platform. "Hmm, the steam doesn't half travel," he said in reference to the thick covering that enveloped the station.

"I think that's fog," said Frank. "That's bizarre, it was like a summer's day in Castletown, and now you can't see the end of your nose in Douglas."

Stan looked at his watch, licking his upper lip and waggling his eyebrows cartoonishly. "Four in the afternoon, young Frank. Must be time for a pint of the Island's finest?"

Frank didn't need asking twice, and they were soon positioned outside the British pub which, in spite of the fog, gave a splendid view over the boats moored in the harbour. They watched a portly gentleman sat topless in a chair on the deck of his boat, waiting patiently for the sun to reappear. All thoughts of an afternoon sail were now forgotten, judging by the beer in his hand.

"You always said you were going to get a boat one day," said Stan.

"True enough," said Frank, smiling wistfully. "Though I think I said I was going to do a lot of things. Sadly, time catches you up. I wanted a quaint little barge to travel across the country, but she always said it was stupid, and boring, the wife, so I never bought one."

"Ah. Unlucky," Stan said, not unkindly.

"I'm not sure if it is old age in general," Frank continued on. "Or this, this... shit inside of me. But I'm feeling vulnerable. I'm afraid that I'm going to lose the desire to do things. Everything I've done in my life has been with one eye on the next thing. When we bought our first taxi, I wanted two. When I bought my first house, I wanted another one — with a bigger garden. Not greedy, mind, just driven to better myself. I'm worried that I'm looking at the final credits scrolling down on the story of my life. I don't like it, Stan."

"We'll buy a boat," said Stan, matter-of-fact. "I don't recall seeing a number two item on the bucket list. We could buy a boat, and seek out adventure on the high seas!"

Frank smiled on one side his mouth, not committing to a full smile but appreciating Stan's efforts. "We'd just end up like that chap over there, most likely, sat on our boat drinking beer with no intention of going anywhere."

"That's not so bad?" Stan offered.

"I'm sorry, Stan. I'll snap out of it. That train journey really brought me back to being a kid, in a nice way. I'm just feeling nostalgic and beginning to realise how fragile life is, that's all."

"All the more reason to enjoy it while you've got it, Frank. Remember my old Aunt Evelyn? She was so obsessed with being ill that we all thought it *made* her ill. It was as if that defined her. You need to see this as a challenge, Frank. One that we're going to get you through," Stan assured him.

"I know, you're right. We'll have a couple of pints and wander up to see Dave and Monty before the practices," replied Frank.

"No practices tonight, I'm afraid," announced the barman, collecting the empties from the outside tables. "Manannán's Cloak has other plans!"

Frank and Stan smiled and nodded like they knew what he was talking about, though they hadn't a clue.

The cheery barman's head was smooth as a baby's bum, while he had the sort of beard small woodland creatures could easily make a home in without your ever being aware. He placed the glasses back on the table and gestured with dramatic effect toward the partially-covered hills in the distance. Like a veteran of the stage, his demeanour changed and his voice lowered an octave or two. "Manannán's Cloak," he told them. "Is the ancient Sea God, Manannán mac Lir, swathing his kingdom in mist to protect it from unwanted visitors."

He was clearly getting into character, much to the frustration of the thirsty punters waiting for a drink. He continued...

"The cloak would roll in from the sea, covering the Island from prying eyes and unwelcome invaders. The grey and purple fog would only lift when our enemies had passed us by."

He paused for further dramatic effect, raising one eyebrow and holding his gaze for slightly longer than was comfortable. Almost on command, the bellowing, deep tone of a fog-horn from the entrance to the harbour reverberated like the beating drum from an invading force. The only thing the skilled orator was missing was a plume of smoke and dramatic explosion, for a magician's exit. Though, in this case, the magician's exit simply meant tending bar once again.

Stan smiled politely till he'd taken their glasses, and he and Frank retreated back through the thirsty hordes, leaving them in their wake as they found a table.

"Was he a bit simple, you reckon?" Stan asked once they were sat.

"Says the fella waving a plastic sword about only minutes ago!" Frank laughed. And then, shrugging his shoulders, said, "I dunno, I quite enjoyed it. Especially the horn at the end. So, anyways, no practice tonight? That's a bit of a nuisance. How many laps do Dave and Monty have to do?"

Stan pulled out his race guide for a look. "Well, they didn't complete a lap last night, and they won't be doing any tonight. They need to do three complete laps before Sunday, so... should be okay?"

Frank frowned. "Sunday? It's Wednesday today, and the races start on Saturday. That means they've only got tomorrow and Friday to complete three laps. Dave said one of the laps has to be a certain time, linked to the third-fastest lap of the other competitors?"

Stan continued to flick the pages. "Yes, at the end of practice week, the organisers look at the entire leaderboard of lap times for every competitor over the course of the week. Any racer wanting to qualify must have at least one lap which is within a-hundred-and-fifteen percent of the third-fastest lap on the overall leaderboard."

"Explain," said Frank.

"Right," said Stan, as if he were suddenly an expert, and having to explain earnestly and patiently to an initiate. "Say the third-quickest qualifying lap overall, from every racer, was a-hundred-and-fifteen miles per hour, yeah? Right, so Dave and Monty would have to complete three laps, and one of them would have to be at least a hundred miles per hour to qualify, and the speed on the other two is not as important as they just need to complete the laps."

"Mmm, I think I get it. Shit, that's going to be tough, especially with a new engine. It's only when you get here and see the scale of the place you realise how hard a lap actually is."

Stan drained his glass, effortlessly, before responding. "Well, if we're not going to watch the bikes, we may as well have a walk around the local hostelries. It's your round, my old friend, and good luck with the hairy tour guide."

With the practice session cancelled, the streets came alive with folk eager to soak up the jovial atmosphere. The locals would often joke that the Island sunk a little each year with the weight of the annual influx, and it wasn't difficult to believe. In the past, visitors had mainly focussed on Douglas. With the ever-increasing popularity of the TT races, however, people were spreading out even more, keen on taking advantage of other picturesque towns in the Island as well. Industrious campsite owners and rugby clubs were happy to accommodate the overflow, but, wherever you went, there was never a hint of trouble — just people eager to share in the magic.

For years, the iconic Bushy's Beer tent, a short walk from the ferry terminal, was the destination of choice. A hefty tent was erected for two weeks of the year to quench the thirst of visitors, and formed the focal point of the TT entertainment. Giant screens would show race footage, and live bands would keep the hordes entertained. Adrenaline was often fuelled by the large crowd of onlookers, and exuberant bikers would succumb to their moment of glory and leave a doughnut-shaped burn-out in the tarmac. The Island's police were exceptionally tolerant, but the moment of extravagance often led to their collars being felt and an expensive visit to the bike shop to buy a new tyre.

Frank leaned on a metal fence that kept the Bushy's drinkers safely away from the busy road. The passing traffic was like a beauty parade of bikers on a constant loop, and made for compelling viewing. A collective cheer would erupt as reward to any biker providing entertainment to the crowd. Frank had zoned out, but the melancholy he felt earlier in the day was this time replaced with a warm sense of appreciation.

The volume from the crowd increased ten-fold, snapping Frank out of his trance, and was followed by a rapturous round of applause.

"What was that?" asked Stan, handing over a plastic beaker of beer.

"A yellow bike just did a wheelie and the girl on the back decided, it would seem, that it would be an even more enjoyable experience with her top off."

"Oh, poor dear, she'll catch cold," remarked Stan.

Frank laughed. "Only a gay man or her father would say that. I bet you don't know where to look with all these men in leather!"

Stan cleared his throat. "I'm sure I hadn't noticed. We should venture over to the fair later," he said, changing the subject. "It's been years since I've been on the dodgem cars, and we can try and win an oversized teddy bear by throwing a bent arrow. I think they've also got those mini motorbikes. We should have a go on them!"

Frank motioned toward the pavement. "Oh, look. There's a two-pound coin on the floor, just there."

Stan twisted his neck before discreetly walking closer. As anybody who's picked up money in a crowd, Stan turned into a character from a black-and-white silent film, overacting every movement. He gave a forced yawn, stretching his arms above his head. As if by magic, he noticed that the lace on his shoe was showing the early stages of wriggling loose. With a final glance over his shoulder, he moved his right foot forward and lowered himself onto his left knee. He pulled at the shoelace and discovered that it didn't actually need adjustment, and, whilst near the floor, discreetly reached for the two-pound coin. It was stubborn, and his fingernails were trimmed neatly, likely making purchase on the coin difficult. He casually reached out for it once more, but it wouldn't move. Undeterred, he made a half-arsed attempt to ruffle his shoelace, once again, before reaching for the coin, this time with both hands. He now had four fingers attached tighter than a pair of pliers, but the bloody thing wouldn't shift. He looked as if he were about to remove his shoe, perhaps to try and hammer the coin loose with its heel.

Stan shook his head, and, in a moment of clarity, looked up at Frank and several other people who were stood over him laughing.

"You bastard, Frank! You knew that it was glued to the tarmac!"

"Guilty as charged," admitted Frank cheerfully. "I saw some other cheapskate doing the same thing while you were at the bar. At least you're going to be famous, though" he said in reference to the camera phones pointed at him. "Come on, your beer's going warm."

Stan rejoined Frank. "That was a dirty trick," he said.

"The best kind," said Frank.

The pair wandered two steps forward and one step back up Douglas Promenade, accompanied by a three-foot teddy bear.

"I knew you could win him," said Frank. "I had faith in you," he said, slurring his words slightly.

"It would have been cheaper to just *buy* a bloody bear. I must have spent thirty quid trying to shoot a pellet gun that'd clearly had the barrel bent to one side," Stan said.

"Sometimes the barrel is bent but the gun still shoots straight," Frank said.

"What the hell are you talking about?" asked Stan.

"I honestly have no idea," Frank said, and they both had to laugh.

Stan clutched his teddy, which he'd name Harold.

Frank had the happy, vacant smile of a man who'd participated in one too many libations. "But, you had a good time, didn't you?"

"I did, old pal, I did. How's your knee?" asked Stan.

"I'd forgotten about that," replied Frank.

"I think your trousers are for the bin, judging by the hole in the knee."

"I was quick, though. I'm going to buy one of those mini motorbikes when I get home," insisted Frank.

"Mmm, you probably shouldn't," advised Stan, reliving the moment of the tumble on his mobile phone. "If you look at this, Frank, when you get to the corner, you're supposed to negotiate it, not pile straight on. You're lucky the policeman had a sense of humour. Still, at least you've had more laps than Dave and Monty!"

"I love you, Stan, you know that. And you, Henry."

"It's Harold," said Stan, taking the arm of the bear and slapping Frank in the face with it. "I love you, too, you daft old bugger."

Harold said nothing, but it was assumed he felt the same.

A young couple sharing a carton of chips smiled at Frank, Stan, and the large teddy as they meandered unsteadily along the promenade. Amongst the three of them, it was unclear who was supporting who.

Stan started to chuckle to himself. "You know I said I'd get you back for the coin incident?"

"... Yes..." replied Frank warily, waiting for the explanation that was sure to follow.

"Well, when you were doing your Joey Dunlop impression earlier, trying to break lap records, I think I may have sent Stella a text from your phone telling her that you'd developed feelings for her... beyond friendship."

"You think!"

"Well, no, I did."

"You bastard! I wondered why she sent me a text calling me a repulsive-looking slob that she wouldn't piss on if I was on fire. You need to call her tomorrow and put her straight!"

"I will, at some point," said Stan. "But we've got a more important issue to worry about."

"What's that?" asked Frank, his head swimming in a not-unpleasant way.

"Who's going to get to sleep with the dopey-looking hairy monster?"

"You can," said Frank.

"Frank, I was talking to Harold!"

chapter seventeen

thursday – Practice Week.

Today's weather brought to you by Radio TT. Dry and bright for large periods of the morning, with bright sunshine in parts. Unfortunately, we're seeing a band of heavy cloud moving in from the west, which may bring outbreaks of rain later this afternoon, which could be heavy at times. We'll keep in touch with the Met Office, but Thursday practice could be in doubt. It's been a challenging week for qualifying times, particularly for the sidecar outfits, whose session was red-flagged on Tuesday.

"Turn that shit off, Monty!" shouted Dave. "Bloody weather! We've got the bike running like a dream and an engine that could get us to over a hundred and five miles per hour average, and the bastard weather looks like it's going to ruin everything."

"Just when we thought the day couldn't get any worse," announced Monty. "Dickhead alert at ten-o'clock."

Harry McMullan sauntered over like he didn't have a care in the world. "Here you go, Dave, I've bought you a doughnut. Well, when I say bought, I mean I found it, actually. Chucked in the bin. Much like your chances in the race?"

McMullan's hand was held out, and Dave nearly took the doughnut before remembering himself. "I'll pass," he said coldly.

"Suit yourself," McMullan said, shrugging for effect, before sending it sailing an inch from Monty's head.

"Leave him, Monty," said Dave. "Put the fire extinguisher down."

"Aw, c'mon, Dave. I could beat him senseless and make it look like an accident?"

"I know you well could," said Dave. "But we need that fire extinguisher in one piece. Use that cucumber by the fridge…"

"The cucumber? But I was going to use that in my sandwich later," Monty protested. "Why the cucumber?"

"It won't leave as many bruises," explained Dave.

"Ah. Good thinking," replied Monty.

"You two are a bit grumpy this morning," said McMullan cheerfully. "I take it you've just heard the weather forecast, then, judging by the radio you've smashed to pieces?"

"I don't know why you're so smug, McMullan," said Dave. "We're all in the same boat."

"*Au contraire*, my tubby friend. You forget that we got two laps in on Monday night. So, whilst the weather isn't ideal, if it means you don't qualify, then, y'know, it's all good. If practice doesn't happen tonight, we only need one lap tomorrow. You pair of clowns need three laps, and there isn't a hope in hell of you getting three laps in tomorrow night. I'm still a bit pissed that you got that engine, but knowing you've got it, but are unable to use it, gives me such a warm, fuzzy feeling inside as you couldn't imagine."

"On second thoughts, Monty," instructed Dave. "We can always buy another extinguisher."

"Temper, temper, boys!" Harry looked over the end of his nose, giving Dave's sidecar a condescending look of disgust. "I may buy this… *thing*… off you boys, seeing as though you won't be needing it. I could stick it in my garden, yeah? Maybe fill it with soil and have a few flowers poking out of it. It'd be good for something then, at least."

"There will be flowers poking out of your arsehole if you don't fuck off!" shouted Dave.

"♫ I'm singing in the rain ♪ ♫ Just singing in the rain ♪" chirped McMullan merrily, as he left them there.

"I could spend days thinking about the best way to hurt him," said Monty.

"Yep, he's got a face you wouldn't tire of slapping with a trout. But he has got a point, though, bastard that he is — and that's if we don't get out tonight, three laps tomorrow is going to be pretty tough."

Monty finally set the fire extinguisher down. "I could've," he said under his breath.

"There's no point hanging about here, Monty," said Dave. "Let's go and buy something for lunch — the greasier the better."

chapter eighteen

Stan sat on the seawall, hunched over a plastic cup full of lukewarm coffee.

"We should have gone to bed when we got in," he said. "That bear scared the hell out of me this morning — I thought I'd brought someone home with me."

"You woke up with fur stuck to your lips," said Frank.

"He was a good kisser, I admit," replied Stan.

They looked out at the ocean, and the waves crashing in.

"My head still hurts," Stan announced. This was yet one in a row of very similar announcements.

"You should keep telling me about your head, Stan. It will make it better if you tell me enough times!" Frank replied. "It was good fun, though, up with Henk and his friends. They're all crazy, but what a bunch of wonderful guys, and that offer was so generous."

Stan knew he should know, but he didn't. "I thought you were drunker than me. So how don't I know what you're talking about?"

"Henk and his friends said that they'd help out with the charity."

Stan bobbed his head slowly. "Ah, I vaguely remember that. Something about a work placement?"

"Exactly! They were going to throw some cash into it, but between them, they've got businesses all over the country — garages, dealerships, and shops. They employ hundreds, and they've said they'll join with us to offer work experience. It won't pay much, but it will certainly give those that want to get back into work some hope. Cash is wonderful, but this gives them longer-term prospects and some workplace skills. I've told Henk and his friends that we're going to take them out for a meal, next week, you know, to say thank-you for everything."

"The least we could do. Now you mention it, I think I may have invited them all to stay with us back home. So, are you going to tell me what we're doing here?" asked Stan. "I must admit this sea breeze is helping me to feel a bit better, but my stomach is in pieces. That kebab probably wasn't the best idea."

"Here we go!" said Frank. "You're going to love this, Stanley."

"Is it, Frank?" asked a short, stout man with a beard ZZ Top would envy.

"It is, and this is Stan. And you must be Andy?"

Andy nodded, handing them some papers. "If you could fill these forms in. Just the usual waivers — you know, if I kill you, you can't sue me, and such — bog standard."

"What the hell are you doing to us?" whispered Stan.

"You'll see. Just sign," said Frank.

"What the hell is a Trike Tour?" asked Stan, observing the logo on the waiver form. "Is a trike not one of them things that children pedal, with the three wheels?"

"It is, my friend," Andy explained. "But it's also," he said, pausing for dramatic effect, "One of *these* magnificent creatures."

With impeccable timing, a black trike with polished alloy wheels pulled into the car park.

"Is that it??" asked Stan, getting suddenly more enthusiastic. "It looks like a three-wheeled, three-seated version of the Batmobile!"

"Pretty cool, right!" said Frank.

Andy gave them a moment to appreciate their steed, before ushering them to a large van parked nearby. "I've got everything you need — gloves, helmet, boots and leathers."

"Hallo, did you say leathers?" asked Stan, with obvious interest.

"Sure," said Andy. "They'll keep you warm. And if the worst happened, they'd give you more protection than your pair of jeans"

"You don't need to convince me, Andy," said Stan. "I've been looking for an excuse to get a set of leathers on for years. I nearly bought a bike last year for that very reason."

A few minutes and they stepped down from the van wearing matching white leathers, carrying white open-faced helmets with black visors. On first glance they looked like the crew of Apollo 13, or, possibly, like they were about to be the ammunition in a circus cannon.

"Looking great, guys," insisted Andy. "You just need to pop these earpieces in, which means we can communicate with each other. I'll let you enjoy the trip, so won't speak too much, but I'll tell you when we're passing through the main parts of the course. We'll be about two hours, and if the weather is nice up the mountain, we'll stop for a photo, but the forecast isn't the best."

Stan and Frank mounted the beast, taking their position in the well-appointed seats raised up behind Andy, the driver.

"Sound-check," said Andy, holding aloft his thumb. With a nod of confirmation from his two passengers, he eased the monster of a bike away from the Douglas Ferry terminal. "Next stop, Quarterbridge, where we'll join the TT course."

Quarterbridge was a premium viewing point; it was close to Douglas, the campsites, and, importantly, had a pub. It was a series of roundabouts connecting Douglas with roads to the south, west, and north of the Island. It was a junction that created difficulty for an inordinate number of racers, as riders would have just negotiated Bray Hill flat out, then onto

Quarterbridge Road equally as quick, before having to brake to a virtual standstill — often on cold tyres — before taking the sharp right-hander onto Peel road towards Braddan Church (another popular viewing spot for spectators). It was one of the slowest points of the course, but one with its unique challenges that would punish even the slightest lapse in concentration.

"Okay, hopefully you're comfortable back there," said Andy. "We're coming up to Braddan Church, and as we progress through, imagine for a moment you're racing through the left then right-hand bend, in front of the grandstands near the church — which would have hundreds of people cheering you on."

The wooden benches were empty apart from a few people watching the traffic pass by. Frank nodded back as the spectators pointed out their impressive trike to their friends and gave a friendly wave. They were doing the speed limit in front of ten men and a dog, and Frank had goosebumps all over, and so he could only imagine the adrenaline the actual racers experienced must have been overwhelming. Frank had seen TV coverage of the racing, but it was impossible to get a genuine feeling for how many twists and turns there were in the course until now.

As soon as they'd hit a straight road, they were navigating another series of bends as they passed through Union Mills.

Andy crackled into their earpieces. "At the top of this hill is Ballagarey, often called Balla*scary* due to the speed in which the right-hander is taken. You really do need balls made of steel to tackle it at full speed."

Stan opened the visor of his helmet. In spite of the cool, refreshing breeze, beads of sweat poured down his face, and it was a face that had taken on a tinge of green.

"You okay?" mouthed Frank.

Stan nodded his head unconvincingly, but it was clear he was in discomfort.

"That's where we watched the practices," said Frank, pointing to their viewing spot from Tuesday evening.

Stan continued to sweat, and it looked like the well-rehearsed delivery from Andy was largely falling on deaf ears in his case. Every bump in the road produced a gurgle from his stomach, and Frank wondered if poor Stan was in danger of losing his lunch, and, if so, which end of Stan it would come out of.

The bike eased to a gentle halt as the traffic lights sat on red. "This is Ballacraine, just less than eight miles from the start line," Andy said, taking advantage of the brief interlude. "If we continued straight on, we'd end up in Peel, but we're turning right to remain on the course." Andy pointed at the house on the opposite side of the road. "You may recall that house? It used to be a pub and was in the classic TT film *No Limit*, with George Formby famously crashing into it, through the front doors. If you haven't seen it, you should. Look behind you, if you can," Andy added. "We have quite the convoy!"

Frank wound his neck and the spectacle behind them was remarkable. A tailback of bikes, three or four abreast, both filled the width of the tarmac, and stretched the length of the road aft of them, like ants grouping up on a jam sandwich. Now his head was turned, he could tune in to the ear-splitting roar.

"A trip around the course is a rite of passage for many visitors fortunate to be accompanied by their own bikes," Andy carried on instructively, obviously relishing the part of tour guide. "There are no speed restrictions on the mountain section of the course — which became one-way over the TT period — but in all other areas of the Island, normal speed limits remain in place for your regular non-racing riders. Whilst most observe the laws of the Island, there are inevitably a small minority who flout the laws and ride considerably quicker than their abilities — sometimes resulting in accident, injury, and worse. This, unfortunately, not only affects those injured but delays the race as well if sections of the course need to be cleaned up before start of the day's racing."

Frank extended his arm and took a selfie of themselves, with their chorus line behind them. The first few bikes raised their thumbs and Stan made his best effort to offer a pained smile for the camera.

The more eager riders jostled for position, and as the lights turned to green they accelerated aggressively, hoping to have a clear road ahead for their lap of the course. Progress from the lights, therefore, was like walking through treacle as every time the vehicle in front moved, the space was filled by those with less patience.

They sat for three cycles of the lights, with Stan looking distressed and clutching his bum on either side in what appeared to be an increasingly desperate effort to keep the cheeks closed.

"Stan?" inquired Frank.

"I'm fine," Stan squeaked. "Actually, maybe not so fine... if we could, ah, perhaps..."

But they were off again.

Frank could feel the phone in the leather pocket vibrating incessantly. It was probably Molly again. He wasn't ignoring her. If anything, she'd been on his mind more than ever over the last few days. She'd love this, he thought. It was difficult to comprehend that the image-conscious, immaculately-dressed woman was once a tomboy who'd doted on him. If there was the prospect of danger, she was in her element; if it involved an engine, so much the better. At least, that's the way it used to be. More than anything, Frank wanted the relationship with his little girl back — but his biggest fear was that it was now too late.

"We're doing about fifty miles an hour," said Andy, once they were back on their way and up to speed. "And we're coming into Sulby Straight, so indulge me once more with your imagination."

Frank's phone was vibrating in his pocket again, but he was paying it no mind at the moment.

Stan's stomach was involved in a summersault routine.

"There's a speed marker at the end of this section, and some of the racers have been clocked going over two-hundred miles per hour. Let that sink in for a moment as we travel through. This isn't a circuit where there are gravel traps or foam barriers every five meters — these are narrow roads, flanked by trees with immovable objects such as lampposts and bus shelters. Travelling through here at that rate must feel like you're moving at light-speed!"

"Are we, ah, due to pull in anytime soon... erm, somewhere? Em... anywhere, actually?" interrupted Stan, shifting uncomfortably in his seat.

"Sure, not a problem," replied Andy. "I was going to take us through Ramsey and then we head up to the mountain. If I can find a safe spot, I'll pull over. Hopefully it will be a good photo opportunity and you can watch some of the bikes passing by. Is that okay with you guys, probably about ten minutes or so? The views up top are stunning."

"Yes, yes!" agreed Stan. "And it needn't be a safe spot."

"A unique aspect of the Island is the ever-changing landscape," Andy said, back to tour-guide mode. "One moment, you're surrounded on all sides by a canopy of trees, which will break periodically to offer a glimpse into the glorious, rolling Manx countryside, and the next, you're in a picturesque seaside town."

"An unsafe spot would do just fine," Stan reiterated, whimpering.

"We're only passing through Ramsey today," said Andy, seemingly oblivious to Stan's circumstance. "But if you get the chance in future, you really should pop back for a visit. We're just about to go through Ramsey Hairpin, and you'll notice that the road changes to one-way traffic between here and the Creg-ny-Baa. Because of this, we may get a few more speeding bikes overtaking. Hopefully we're ahead of the adverse weather coming in, so try and enjoy the scenery at top — it's wonderful."

The mountain section of the course rose majestically from Ramsey at sea level, up to the Island's only mountain, and highest point — Snaefell, at 2,034 ft. Fortunately, the heavy covering of cloud to the north of the Island had yet to make landfall, so, as Andy had promised, they had an uninterrupted view of the picturesque yet rugged landscape — though Stan was in no condition to notice.

"It's pretty special up here!" said Frank. Then, looking over at Stan, said, "Yes, anytime you might be able to make that stop. It's just... there appears to be some urgency in the matter."

Stan squeaked in agreement.

Green hills overlapped each other in whichever direction you looked. A vibrant yellow from the sporadic patches of gorse bushes was complemented by a peppering of white sheep scouring the terrain for an easy meal. It was breathtaking, so much so that Stan, dumbfounded by the beauty of this place, forgot his discomfort if only for a moment.

"We're going to pull in over there, on the left," said Andy, "Just before the sharp right-hand bend."

Ironically, considering Stan's current predicament, their photo opportunity was at a part of the course called Windy Corner.

The instant the bike came to a stop, the helmet was off and Stan was gone...

***

Stan had no firm plan at this stage, but his stomach was making noises like a volcano about to erupt and Stan wanted that eruption to be on his terms. He walked as fast as he could with his buttocks still clenched, his thighs pressed together, and his lower legs motoring quicker than the passing bikes. "Ow, ow, ow," he said on repeat.

Fortunately, there was not a soul to be seen. He quickly navigated a small wooden stile into a field surrounded by an ornate stone wall, making sure his travelling companions were out of sight as he began to pull at the gloves.

"Come on!" he screamed in frustration, pulling at the Velcro, dancing on the spot like a madman at a disco.

He eventually released his right hand, and fought a battle with the left-hand glove which proved even more elusive. He gripped it and pulled with every ounce of strength before his hand finally came free... with such energy that his hand recoiled, smashing him full-force on the bridge of the nose.

"Bastard!" screamed Stan, as a thin trickle of blood seeped down his face.

The zip on the leathers was secured by a button at the top, but Stan's hands were freezing from the bike ride and the howling wind, making purchase on the fastening difficult. He pulled at the leather suit like a lunatic escaping from a straitjacket. His vision was blurred by a flood of tears from the whack on his nose, and this did nothing to further the cause. The button eventually burst, and he was able to pull the zip down to his waist. As instructed, he only wore underpants and a t-shirt, so the bottom half of the suit fell to the ground with little resistance. Stan crouched down a split-second before the volcano burst to life in an explosion of biblical proportions.

***

"What the hell was that noise!" shouted Frank.

"That's the new Ducati," said Andy, pointing at the gleaming red machine speeding by.

"That sounds amazing!" said Frank.

***

Stan was in rapture; the relief was instant, although he was unsure what to do next. He pulled a clump of grass behind him but there wasn't enough to create sufficient density to be able to wipe effectively. He pulled the insurance waiver from his pocket and considered that for a moment, before dismissing it.

He scoured the field for inspiration. He noticed clumps of brown wool flapping in the wind, secured to the barbed wire that ran along the perimeter of the stone wall. He looked at the wall above where he crouched. Fortunately, the wire that prevented sheep from escaping may now come to his rescue. He stretched his arm up and began to pluck like it was a toilet-paper tree. He was hopeful, but the strands simply parted whenever he applied any pressure. He remained crouched as he tried to reach out for another patch of wool. It was just out of reach and he was reluctant to stand without wiping. He shuffled his feet but there was virtually no grip on the damp grass and his feet gave way causing him to fall face first. He lay on the ground and knew there was only one solution: his t-shirt would have to make the ultimate sacrifice.

With the paperwork for the job sorted out, he smiled to himself, and began to raise himself up into a more dignified position... and found he had an audience. "Hello?" he said, startled.

A fiendish-looking sheep with entirely too many horns stared directly at him. Judging by its colouring, it might very well have been the source of the wool he'd just used in an attempt to conclude his business.

The sheep, for its part, looked wholly displeased.

"Nice sheep?" asked Stan, tentatively, although he had no idea what sort of sheep this was, exactly, staring him down, as he'd never seen one quite like this.

It began making aggressive gestures, and Stan had no desire to hang about for an introduction. It was soon joined by another, and then another, and Stan was now faced with a dizzying number of aggressive-looking horns he didn't care to stop and count. He leapt to his feet and clutched the trousers of his leather suit. The trousers were still round his ankles, and he did a combination of a hop and a run as he stooped to pull them up to his waist. The first sheep didn't even have to break into a trot to inflict its first assault.

"Help me!" screamed Stan. "I'm being attacked!"

The animal was inquisitive and placed its cold nose on Stan's bum. "Nice sheep?" he said again, in his calmest voice. But before waiting for an answer, he gathered himself up, once again, and hurdled the wooden stile like Daley Thompson.

He had to let go of the trousers to cushion his fall with his hands as he landed on the other side of the wall, out of harm's way. He stood with the leather trousers crumpled at his feet, and, as he'd found another use for his t-shirt, only had his (formerly) white underpants on.

"Are we going to have a problem here?" said a marshal who'd turned up in response, presumably, to his cries for help. "One blast on this radio and the police will be here in minutes."

"No," said Stan, struggling for breath. "But thank goodness you're here. I've been... I've been assaulted by devil creatures. Just there!"

"Those are Loaghtan sheep," she said flatly.

"I'll probably just, ah, go... then... shall I?" said Stan, pulling his suit back up, attempting to restore as much dignity as he could muster, which, it turnt out, was not an awful lot.

The marshal, staring Stan down in much the same way as the Laughton devil-sheep, kept her radio in hand, thumb hovering at the ready, as he made his exit.

***

"Thanks for your help, Frank. I could have been killed!" said Stan, upon his return.

"I thought it best to leave you to your own devices, surely?" said Frank.

"Yes, well..." said Stan.

"Well, what?" asked Frank, and, then, after turning round, "What the hell happened to you??"

Frank had been using his camera to record the splendour of the panoramic view, but he couldn't resist taking several shots of Stan in his current state as this was, after all, what friends were for.

"I needed the toilet, but there was no paper, and then..."

"And then what?" Frank asked, not overly concerned with the answer, happily snapping a few more photos of Stan instead.

"Well, let's just say things got a little woolly!" Stan said in angry exasperation.

"Alright, alright, calm down, mate," Frank said, before taking one last picture. "No need to get shirty."

There's no way are we getting out," said Dave.

The adverse weather that had threatened for most of the afternoon now gave the evening light an angry, bruised effect. The practice session for the solo bikes had commenced on time, but the sidecars were scheduled for later in the evening.

Like most of the impatient sidecar crews, Dave and Monty looked longingly toward the sky, but it was inevitable as they felt the first few drops of rain falling on their faces.

"For fuck's sake!" screamed Dave.

The public-address system gave its very familiar *BING-BONG*, announcing that the clerk of the course had an announcement to make. Dave had already started pushing his machine; he knew what was coming.

"That's us, Monty. The dream is over for another year. There is not a snowball in hell's chance that we're going to get out for three laps tomorrow night."

Harry McMullan was also furious. He had two laps under his belt, but he needed the valuable lap time to fine-tune the set-up of the bike. He forced his way past the young spectators who were eager to add his signature to their caps and shirts.

"Piss off," he said, marching through them. He stopped and turned on a six-pence. The children could be forgiven for thinking he might be coming back to apologise, but he marched straight through them once again.

"That's the quickest that piece of shit is going to go this TT week!" McMullan said, pointing at Dave, who was still pushing his bike, and then stomped off in a sulk.

Dave didn't break his stride and simply extended a one-finger salute.

"Oops, sorry about that, kids. I didn't see you there," said Dave. "Would you like me to sign that?" he asked, stopping and pulling a pen from his pocket.

"Not really," said the oldest of the three kids. "But you may as well finish, seeing as though you've started."

"You'd do well to steer clear of Harry McMullan," said Dave, providing the kids with some fatherly, sage advice. "He's a miserable git, and leaves a trail of nasty in his wake."

"Yeah," said one of the children, a beautiful young girl with sun-bleached blonde hair and an angelic face. "Yeah, he's a dickhead."

Dave was shocked to hear that sort of language issued forth from such a pretty little face. Shocked, but proud.

"Then why—?"

"We get twenty quid on eBay for his signature," the older boy explained, and, right afterwards and with interest, "Are you famous, then?"

"Just you wait, lad," said Dave with a grin. "Just you wait and see."

chapter nineteen

friday – Final Day of Practices.

Today's weather brought to you by Radio TT. It's been a mixed bag for weather on the Island this week, but it's going to be dry with long sunny spells and temperatures due to touch mid-twenties in parts. As we turn to the evening, it should be very pleasant conditions for the final practice session. Race Control has announced a change to the practice schedule, with the sidecars due to head out first, at six-twenty p.m.

Dave groaned in pain. "I think we need more oil, Monty. It just doesn't feel right."

"I've just done that. What's wrong, overheating?"

"I think so. Maybe I just need to top-up with water. Try the oil first and we'll take it from there."

"The handlebars are a bit loose."

"Good point, don't be shy with the oil, that's the bit I always miss."

"Okay, but, Dave, I can't get the angle to get stuck into it."

"You'll just need to climb on, Monty. And take your time, if it burns we could be in real trouble for tonight."

"I'm struggling to get the lid off, Dave."

"Monty, do I need to do everything? Improvise! Use your mouth."

"I am, I've just nearly broken a bloody tooth and I've got it all over my face."

"Stop your whingeing, Monty and climb on. And they're not handlebars, they're love handles — the ladies love them."

Monty straddled Dave's back. "I think these swimming trunks are a little neat, Dave."

"Get the cream on the cheeks, Monty — you don't want me getting sunburn down there when we've got an important race tomorrow."

"Preparation going well?" asked Frank, as they approached the awning.

Monty looked up and cream was now running down his chin.

"I think we've interrupted the boys at an awkward time," said Frank, chuckling to Stan.

Monty and Dave were both naked apart from swimming trunks — trunks which would be best described as modest, bordering on offensive.

"Lovely shorts," remarked Stan.

"For some reason, they seem to keep the autograph-hunters away," said Dave. "The bike is running like a dream, so we've decided to have a bit of rest and recuperation ahead of the practice session."

"It's great that they've brought the practice session forward," said Frank. "Are you confident for three laps?"

"Nope," replied Dave immediately. "But we'll give it a go. You guys couldn't do me a favour?"

"Of course," replied Stan. "What do you need?"

"Move a bit to the left. You're in my sun, old son," said Dave.

Frank and Stan shuffled to the left. "We just wanted to drop by and, you know, wish you the best of luck."

"Where are you watching?" asked Monty. "I've got a couple of spare pit passes if you want to watch there?"

"Thanks, but I think we're going to go to that place where Henk took us the other night. It was a great spot," said Stan.

"I'll wave as we go past," said Dave. "Anyway, don't mean to be rude, chaps, but Monty, can you finish up with the sun cream, and while you're there, that knot in my shoulder isn't going to work itself out."

"Are you not going to answer that?" asked Stan.

"No, it's a private number. Probably Molly again," replied Frank.

"You're not speaking with her?"

"No. Well, yes. I mean, yes, but not right now. She's getting on my case. She means well, though. She's been different the last few days."

"Different how?"

"It's hard to explain. She's just being, well, *nice*. Like the Molly of old."

"That's not good?" asked Stan.

"It's very good. I'm enjoying it, but she's just been getting on my case a bit over the last couple of days like I said."

The Island was resplendent with the absence of cloud. The bright sunshine brought a happy glow to the fields and the cattle looked idyllic, like they'd been glued in position to cement the image of tranquil countryside. Frank and Stan joined the railway line at Quarterbridge, walking along where the old tracks had once been — and was now a lovely walking path — with the intention of taking a longer, but more leisurely stroll to their viewing spot. The early stages of the railway line were largely under the cover of trees, with the River Dhoo meandering gently alongside. Two backpacks were filled with essentials and they'd acquired a radio to listen to the coverage of the practice session.

"Why's she been getting on your case?" asked Stan.

Frank pointed out a grey heron on the riverbank, but his deflection tactic failed.

"Frank?"

"It's nothing. I just told her something about my treatment that she didn't like."

"What about your treatment?"

Frank picked up a large twig and threw it on the water, watching as it floated downstream.

"I've refused treatment."

"What? You're joking, of course?"

"I'm not joking, no. The doctor gave me all the available options and I've said I'll let him know when I get back home."

"That's lunacy!" said Stan, getting more animated. "I can see why Molly is getting on your case!"

"Stan, I know you care, but this is why I didn't tell you. It's why I wasn't going to tell anyone. I hadn't meant to tell Molly, but her being nice and all just caught me off guard and it'd slipped out. Stan, I'll know what I need to do when I get back. It's not as if anything is going to change over the next week, right? So promise me we can leave it at that. If it turns out I'm being nagged by everyone, then I'll end up just keeping things to myself again, yeah?"

Stan looked down at the ground, as if he were studying the dirt intently. "Bloody sod," he said, under his breath.

"What?" asked Frank.

"Okay, I promise," Stan said after a few moments. "Please don't block us out, though, Frank, because people care. Wait, what are you smiling at? I'm being serious here!"

"I know, mate. Molly told me that her mum has kicked the fitness instructor into touch."

"And you're happy? You don't want her back, do you?"

Frank looked offended. "I'd rather massage baby oil onto Monty and Dave's naked torsos after they've completed the three laps, in this heat, than go back to Helen. I suppose I just receive some perverse pleasure in her having a hard time. Call it *schadenfreude*, I guess."

"Why?" Stan asked.

"Because that's what it's called."

"Oh. Anyway, it's understandable, I suppose, you should feel that way. I wonder what happened on her end, though.

Maybe she finally realised she prefers geriatric blokes who're past their sell-by date, rather than a toned Latvian Adonis?"

"Thanks, Stan, you know how to make someone feel good. If you want, I can ask if she'll put a word in for you with Boris."

Stan looked as if he were actually considering the suggestion for a moment, but then shook his head. "Come on, Frank," he said. "We need to pick the pace up, we've got a few miles to go."

They pushed on through the Manx countryside, with two cans of beer opened to refresh the intrepid travellers. The perception of just how far they'd travelled, however, was somewhat confusing as great swathes were similar. "I remember this cricket club," said Stan. "Is this not where we parked the other night?"

Frank flicked the switch on the radio and the unmistakable enthusiasm of the commentators indicated the start of the practice session was imminent.

"We're going to have to run!" said Frank.

"I'm not running. If I run, I shall perspire," replied Stan, trying his best to sound posh. "And a gentleman does not perspire!"

"But we'll miss the start!" Frank protested.

"Frank, you're past your expiry date — no offence — and I'm chronically unfit. We're not running. There's no way an ambulance could reach us here, and do you really want to carry me over your back? Or, me, you?"

"Okay, point taken," said Frank, taking a mouthful from his can. "We're not exactly athletes, hairy muff, but let's ramp it up a notch?"

They were within sight of the wooden gate that spanned the width of their path, ahead.

"There it is," said Frank pointing just further on. "We turn right after that, and we're there. Listen, I can hear them coming!"

The monstrous roar of screaming engines once again disturbed the still, evening air, causing the hair on the back of their necks to stand to attention. The impending arrival of the first bike on the road felt like a summer storm; even though they couldn't see it yet, they could feel it in the air, sense the change in pressure.

The wind seemed to develop a chill, suddenly, and the lads waited in anticipation for the first bike to strike in like a crack of lightning.

"I love this!" shouted Stan, as they ran to the familiar piece of rope up against the road, and, once there, embracing it like an old friend. This piece of rope, sturdy as it may have been, was the only thing separating the fans from the racers, and Stan and Frank clutched it tightly with excitement.

Frank pressed the radio close to his ear. "I think they just said Number Thirty-Two is away?" He stuck his finger in his other ear, trying in vain to drown out the roar of thunder passing a few feet from where they stood.

"Thirty-Nine, Forty, Forty-Two — they're away! Go on, Dave, go on, Monty!" they screamed, jumping like teenage girls at a One Direction concert.

"Easy, remember your condition!" Stan shouted.

"What condition??" Frank yelled back.

"I don't know!" Stan replied. "You've never told me!"

"Well, then!" Frank shouted, and, with that, they carried on screaming and jumping like the aforementioned teenaged girls.

Any other sporting spectacle of this magnitude would have hundreds of people jostling for position at a prime viewing spot like this. They were touching-distance away from bikes passing in a blur at 150 mph. It was exhilarating, and they were on their own with only a pocket radio to keep them company.

"I feel like I'm going to shit myself again!" announced Stan. "And it's not kebab-related this time!"

You didn't have a moment to think, to breathe — even blinking became an unwelcome distraction.

"Any second now!" shouted Frank, as Outfit Number Forty passed quickly but safely through.

Frank and Stan stared at the brow of the hill like hungry dogs by the dinner table.

"That's Forty-Three and Forty-Four!" said Frank.

Several more outfits made their swift arrival — and just-as-swift departure — but Dave and Monty were not among them.

"Where the hell are they??" said Frank.

Stan took the radio and listened intently, but there was no mention of Number Forty-Two.

More of the higher numbers came into view on the road, and then passed by. Frank checked his phone to see if Dave had texted with any problems, but there was nothing.

The road fell quiet, which revealed how loud their radio was. There was always a delay in information from around the course, filtering back to the commentary box.

They heard:

> *Outfit Number Forty-Two has pulled into Quarterbridge to make adju–*

... but the sound of the commentator on the radio was drowned out as Dave and Monty burst into view in a glorious blur of blue and yellow.

Frank and Stan waved their arms furiously, and just as they reached the dip in the road, Dave's head bobbed, and he managed a wave in return as he overtook the outfit that was on the road in front of them.

"Holy shit!" shouted Stan. "They're bloody motoring there, that was amazing! Turn that thing on your phone so we can watch when they go through the checkpoints!"

Dave and Monty were on a charge, but the delay at the start of their lap had severely hampered them. They soon broke the timing beam at Glen Helen, and, although it was only practice week, the timings at the top of the leaderboard were impressive. This put additional pressure on those further down the rankings — including Dave and Monty — and the lap time of the all-important, third-quickest qualifying lap would have been on all the racers' minds.

Stan's knuckles were white from gripping the rope so tightly. "I don't think I've ever felt this nervous! And I bet Dave is taking it in his stride — probably singing to himself! Does the lap time look good?"

"I've no idea," replied Frank. "I'm not really sure how to interpret what I'm looking at. If they stopped at Quarterbridge, then I'd imagine that it won't be that quick, but at least it'll be one of the three laps completed. If the bike holds out, they've got at least two more laps if they can get out before the session closes. Hopefully one of those laps will be quick."

The brief lull in traffic was burst in spectacular style with the arrival of the lower-numbered outfits on view in front of Frank and Stan. Their arrival meant that Dave and Monty would likely be in the vicinity of the start line and at completion of their first lap of the week. Like a child on a long car journey, Stan pestered Frank to know if it'd arrived.

"No," said Frank. "But I don't think the mobile data is particularly good here."

Frank held the phone aloft, walking up and down the length of the rope barrier, hoping he could find a signal that had penetrated the dense canopy of trees.

"Has it worked?" asked Stan.

"Only I wouldn't know, would I, as it's above my head," Frank replied.

Stan stood on his toes to get a better look, but then dropped back down. "Hang on, I've just had a thought," he said.

"Did you?" Frank teased.

"It happens sometimes!" said Stan. "The thing of it is," he continued. "Even if it has got better signal up there, it's of no bloody use to us if we can't see it. There's nothing for it, then — you'll have to climb on my shoulders."

"You must be bloody joking!" said Frank. "If we're not capable of running a few hundred yards, what makes you think we're circus performers all of a sudden?"

"Well I said I had a thought. I didn't say it was a good one, did I?" replied Stan with a shrug.

Frank hit the refresh button and slowly the updated lap times appeared. "They've completed a lap!" said Frank, "Eighty-two-point-six-seventy-eight miles per hour!" he shouted. "It's well off the pace, but at least that's one lap marked off!"

For fear of losing signal, Frank didn't move a muscle and they once again focussed their attention on the right-hander at the top of the road. Never did they think they would spend so much time utterly fascinated by staring at a tree — or for the bikes to come round it, at least.

"It's quite a lovely tree, that," Stan offered, as there was not much else to say at the moment.

"It is," agreed Frank.

The marshals moved their heads, and the sudden increase in decibel level indicated the arrival of the next wave. Dave and Monty came first into view, and were visibly quicker than the bikes around them. Dave was either being unsociable, or his concentration was absolute, as he passed like a bullet discharged from a pistol. There was no wave this time, but the lads didn't seem to mind.

"Shit! He's moving quicker than a scalded cat!" said Stan, dancing on the spot like a young child that's got to pee. "They're going to do this, Frank!" he said. And, then, turning to Frank for confirmation, "They're going to do this??"

"Do they need to stop for fuel?" asked Frank. "Because surely that'll slow them down, if they do?"

"No," Stan assured him. "Monty said they'll be good with the one tankfull for three laps, and that the tyres should also hold out okay as well. So, no pit stops. We just need to hope that whatever happened on the opening lap, whatever that might've been, doesn't happen again."

Such was the progress the boys were making that Chris Kinley gave them a special mention as they advanced through Glen Helen. Frank and Stan watched the app on the phone through closed fingers — willing them to make it to the next timing beacon. They were safely indicated through Ramsey and began the climb up the mountain section, which must have afforded a magnificent view with the glorious weather conditions if they weren't too deep in concentration to notice.

"Come on, Dave," said Stan. He couldn't settle, struggling for something to do with his hands.

"I bet you don't get this feeling watching the F-One," said Frank.

Stan nodded his head. "I know what you mean, this is a different league. Most of the guys doing this don't have pots of cash or a team of mechanics — it's just pure racing. It's truly wonderful. Imagine trying to explain this feeling to anyone else who wasn't here — it can't be done. I guarantee we'll be here next year, and with a load of people who want to experience it for themselves."

"You're optimistic about my prognosis," said Frank, laughing.

"We will be here!" insisted Stan.

"How long is there left of the session?" asked Frank.

"Ten minutes or so," replied Stan, looking at his watch. "Shit, this is going to be really tight."

Chris Kinley was reaching fever pitch on the radio as the close of the session drew in. He knew how important the lap time was for all concerned, and that, for many, their hopes could easily be dashed for another year. Frank and Stan listened intently to the commentary:

Just a reminder folks, that after this session we've got a full schedule for the solo bikes. That's outfit Number Forty-Two — Dave Quirk and Shaun Montgomery — passing the start line and it looks like they're slowing. That's a real shame as they're one of the teams still on two laps, I think. I'll wait for them to come up the return lane and see what the problem was. Tim in the tower, can you shout out a lap time for Number Forty-Two for me?"

Yes, Chris. Number Forty-Two, their first lap was eighty-two-point-six-seventy-eight, and their second lap, bearing in mind they were slowing coming down the return lane, was nevertheless a quite impressive one-oh-one-point-four-three-eight. I can confirm that they have only completed two laps.

Thanks, Tim. And I'm here with Dave. Dave, you've got your team looking at the bike. Now, you pulled in on the first lap, is it a recurrence of that problem?

Dave remained on the bike and now had a microphone pressed into his face. Two mechanics worked furiously on the front fairing, but they shook their heads in frustration, forcing the front down.

"I think so, Chris," Dave said in answer to the question. "The front fairing came loose on the first lap. We pulled in and we thought we'd fixed it, but coming over the mountain it came back again — something must have broken. We were off the pace, so that's us I suppose. We'll just call it a day and look forward to next year."

"That's a real shame, Dave. I don't know about you being off the pace," said Chris Kinley. "With that last lap time, you would have qualified. Tony Dearie and Harry McMullan are third-quickest, and with your time, you would have been right quick enough, no problem."

"You're fucking kidding me?? Why am I sat here, like a lemon, then, talking to you, when I could be fixing the bike???"

Dave jumped off the bike and began attacking the front fairing. He didn't care if it looked pretty; he just needed it to hold in place, safely, for the final lap. After not very long at all, he knelt down, gripped it, and said, "Right. That bugger is going nowhere fast. Chris, how long have we got left?"

Kinley raised his hand, indicating one minute, meaning the gate would soon close and that would be the last opportunity to get out on the bike.

Dave jumped aboard the bike and hit the starter button. The engine turned over, but it wouldn't spark back into life. Dave jumped up and down as he tried once again, hoping to shake back into life whatever was causing the problem.

Chris Kinley pointed out the marshal, who was preparing to close the gate.

"Fuck!"

Dave tried once more, but the engine wouldn't fire into life.

"Give me a push!" he screamed at anyone stood nearby. His two mechanics ran behind and furiously pushed as Dave did everything he could.

"Quicker!" shouted Dave.

Kinley, who was live on air, dropped his microphone and ran behind them, giving them an extra burst of speed. They were reaching the perimeter wall when the engine burst mercifully back into life and they eased back onto the circuit before the gate closed. Dave glanced over his shoulder to check for traffic, before accelerating up Glencrutchery Road for the final qualifying lap.

"Sorry for the silence," Chris said into his mic. "I dropped my microphone helping the lads jumpstart a stalled machine. Amazing scenes here, as outfit Number Forty-Two has made it away with five seconds to spare. Go on, Dave and Monty! Fantastic scenes!"

Dave kept his head down on the final lap. The bike hadn't missed a beat and they'd hit every apex. It wasn't the time for heroics; they had a lap time that should be sufficient to qualify. If they pushed too hard, they could make a stupid mistake or risk a mechanical failure. He was relaxed, and for the first time really believed they could truly qualify.

"Keep 'er steady," Dave said to himself, over and over. He tucked himself in as they hurtled down the notoriously rapid Cronk-y-Voddy Straight. A flash of colour passed him on the right side, completely disorientating him. For an instant, he thought he'd clipped the kerb and was in the process of flipping over, but, as it turnt out, it was another outfit had darted past them like they were standing still.

Dave's heart raced; he thought they were the final outfit out on track, so being overtaken at that pace scared the hell out of him. He took a deep breath and composed himself, but before the outfit in front disappeared from view, he caught sight of Harry McMullan taking the opportunity to raise his middle finger up behind his back.

Dave resisted every urge in his body to chase him down. He knew they were significantly quicker. And, besides, he couldn't let his ego get in the way — he just had to bring her home.

McMullan and Dearie were currently third quickest, but Dave knew that if they increased their time on this lap, he and Monty could likely be pushed out of the qualifying places. Dave didn't want to dwell on this. He couldn't influence what they did, and just had to focus on what he could control. If anything, he rolled off the throttle a little as his heart was still thumping out of his chest.

The temporary fix of the front fairing held firm, and Dave brought Monty and the bike back in one piece. As he rode up the return lane, he had no idea if he'd qualified, but did he care?

Damn right, he did!

The first person he saw was Chris Kinley, who was still live on-air, interviewing Harry McMullan. He cut McMullan short for a moment and held up his clipboard where he'd written:

You've done it by .183 mph!

Chris patted him on the back as Dave leaned over to Monty to deliver the news. A wave of emotion rushed over him and his eyes welled up with tears of relief.

"We've fucking done it, Monty! We've only gone and done it!"

chapter twenty

the beer tent on Douglas Promenade was busy earlier in practice week, but with the races starting the following morning, the place was completely heaving.

"They didn't have champagne, only lager. And warm lager, at that!" said Stan, returning from the bar. "Are you okay, Frank? You look... well, you like you're either in pain or having an orgasm?"

"Just contented," said Frank. "Lager?" he asked, taking his beer.

"Stella," said Stan. "It's all they had, I just said."

"What about Stella?" Frank said, only half-listening.

"Stella Artois. The lager," Stan explained.

"Ah. Right. Thanks, Stan. Sorry, lost in thought. What a day today, yeah? That was amazing. I really didn't think they were going to do it. The commentator sounded like he was going to rupture something, he was so excited! Dave just texted me back, by the way. Says he's going to get his head down early."

Frank's phone rang, and he stared at it, confused.

"Ah, it's a phone," Stan said, teasing him. "That ring you're hearing? They do that sometimes."

"Do they?" Frank said, taking the ribbing like a good sport. "I never knew."

"Is that Molly again?" asked Stan. "Did she ever manage to get hold of you?"

"I did phone her back, yeah," replied Frank. "Said we'd have a good talk about things when I get back. But, no, this is someone calling from a private number, so I can't imagine it's Molly. Probably someone trying to sell me life insurance, although I'm not sure they'd give me a quote at the moment!"

"Hmm," said Stan.

"Yes, hello," said Frank, picking up the call. He closed his eyes to concentrate, and attempted to filter out the noise of the rock band performing thirty feet away, but realised it was a battle he was never going to win. He motioned to Stan for them to move to the far end of the car park on which the tent stood.

"Sorry, I couldn't hear you. You'll need to start again," he said, once they were clear. "Right... Yes, this is Frank."

Stan looked on, concerned.

"Stella gave you my number?" Frank asked the caller.

Who is it?" Stan mouthed, and Frank shrugged his shoulders and shook his head.

Frank went quiet as he listened carefully.

"Look, who the hell is this??" he said, finally. "Hello? Hello?" And, then, to Stan, "The fucker hung up on me!"

"That sounded serious, who on earth was it?" asked Stan.

Frank took a mouthful of his drink and shook his head again.

"I'm not sure, Stan. Some bloke with a foreign accent. Stella had given him my number, apparently."

Stan rolled his eyes. "Let me guess," he said. "Another happy customer she's managed to piss off?"

"No, not this time," Frank said, gravely. "He didn't give me a name, but he was a less-than-pleasant sort. His accent was thick, and he spoke so quickly it was difficult to keep up with him. But he gave me the indication — well, he actually said straight out, near as I could tell — that Lee was thieving scum and he'd only left Ireland before people caught up with him."

Stan paused for a moment to digest the information. "Lee?" he said incredulously. "It doesn't make sense. The guy's a bloody hero! He stopped that robbery, after all, and just look what he's done for the charity, raising all that cash in only a few days."

"Shit, Stan. The cash. What about all the cash?" said Frank.

"The cash is fine," replied Stan. "The money is in the office safe, and Stella has got the only key. If he can break into that safe or he manages to get the key off Stella, then he deserves the cash inside."

"We can't have misjudged the guy that much?" said Frank. He took another mouthful of his beer and replayed in his mind his interactions with Lee. "You know, this could be nothing but a load of rubbish. We can't just go and accuse the guy of something he hasn't done. He's been kicked on the streets for months and the last thing he needs are his new colleagues accusing him of being a thief."

"It's Friday!" exclaimed Stan suddenly.

Frank looked at him, unsure of what point he was trying to make.

"Friday, Frank! Stella will have put the wages for the part-time drivers in the safe!" explained Stan. "Frank, I'm not sure we can take the risk on this. With the money from the charity and the wages, there'll probably be about thirty thousand in that safe!"

Frank shook his head and picked up his phone. "Oh, Stan. What if we've made a giant mistake on this one? What if Lee *is* a thief? Fuck, fuck, fuck! I need to phone Stella and let her know, at least warn her of the possibility."

The two of them walked through the fairground, toward the middle section of the promenade, where it was a little more sedate, and so quieter.

"Stan, I'll do this on speakerphone so you can hear what's being said on both ends," said Frank.

Like phoning most taxi offices, it rang continuously, with no one picking up.

"It's Friday night, they must be busy," offered Stan. "Try her mobile?"

Frank rang her mobile. "Hello," came a gruff voice.

"Stella, it's Frank and Stan. Right. I've got you on speakerphone, luv."

"You two can fuck right off," she said, before hanging up.

"Did she just hang up on us?" said Frank.

"She just hung up on us," said Stan. "Do we need to remind Stella who pays her wages?"

"You can, if you like," replied Frank. "Personally, I'm not that brave. And you must remember my condition."

"And what condition is that again?" asked Stan.

"Extreme cowardice," said Frank. I'm not that brave enough to go toe-to-toe against Stella — even when there's seventy miles of water between us."

"Ah. That one," replied Stan. "Well, if you don't at least try her again, we may not have a pot to piss in very soon."

"I'll try her again, shall I?" Frank said.

"What is it you lot want?" Stella's voice came over speakerphone, as warm and welcoming as ever. "Only I'm really very busy at the moment."

Frank thought it best to take a conciliatory approach. "Sorry, we just tried the work number and it rang and rang. Are you really very busy?"

"At the moment? No, not especially," Stella said, and then made an audible sucking-in noise — the all-too-familiar sound of her taking a long drag off a cigarette.

"I thought you just said—?" Frank ventured.

"I've got Susie in helping," replied Stella.

"Ah, good. That's nice. You sound like you're talking with an echo?"

"I'm in the toilet! Having a shit, if you must know!" Stella replied, with sufficient volume over speakerphone that the elderly couple unfortunate enough to be enjoying an evening stroll along the promenade nearby now surely also knew.

"But I just heard you smoking?" said Frank.

"I smoke when I shit!" said Stella. "Get over it! It helps me to relax, dunnit!"

"Thanks, Stella, I'm happy you're relaxed," said Frank, nearly retching.

"Easy, Frank," Stan said encouragingly, patting Frank on the back.

"Damn straight I'm relaxed!" came the relaxed reply. "And was that Stan I just heard? Stan, you can fuck right off!"

"Lovely to hear your voice as well," Stan replied.

"Look, I'll keep this brief," said Frank.

"Thank Christ!" Another long sucking-in of air.

"Look, have you seen Lee lately?"

"In the women's loo? I should hope not!" Stella responded. "Is there something about him I should know about? Is he a stalker of beautiful women such as myself??"

"I meant in general," Frank replied, as placidly as possible, so as to maintain her relaxed state.

"Oh. Shame, then," said Stella. "No. His mate, the old git, has been in looking for him. He was sat in your office for about three hours, staring at the wall. Probably dribbling. One of the drivers said they saw Lee near Lime Street Station, earlier, though."

Frank felt his shoulders drop. "Stella, did he seem okay when you spoke to him last?"

"What? I've not spoken to that idiot more than once," she said. "Why do you ask?"

"No reason," said Frank, unconvincingly. "Did you put the wages in the safe, by any chance?"

"Frank, it's Friday!" she admonished him. "When have I not put the bloody wages in the bloody safe on a bloody Friday! What's going on??"

"Stella, I've just had a phone call to say Lee might not be quite the knight in shining armour that we thought he was."

"I soddin' well told you that, didn't I, you bloody pair of gormless wankers. But does anyone ever listen to Stella? No, they bloody well don't! As soon as I've finished up here, I'm getting that old bloke and hanging him up by his bollocks. He must know where Lee is. When I get some information out of him, I'll let you Dickhead Twins know."

"Don't be daft, Stella," said Stan. "If he knew where Lee was, why would he be hanging about the office? Anyway, why are you so keen to find Lee?"

"You mean besides what you just said? Because he's got the bloody safe key!" Stella replied. "He told me he was putting some cash in that they'd been given over the last couple of days. And I assumed he'd just forgotten to give me the key back."

"Has he taken the cash from the safe?" asked Frank, tentatively.

"How the hell would I know? He's got the bloody key, so I can't very well open it to bloody check, now can I?"

"Why did you give him the key?" ventured Stan, rather bravely.

"Don't start that with me, Stan, or I'll smash your bollocks in as well. You told me he was working for you, and he's been poncing around here like he owns the bloody place!"

"*Shit, shit, shit,*" mouthed Frank. "Look, Stella, me and Stan are going to get a plane home in the morning. Don't call the police just yet, this could be all a big misunderstanding and nothing more, yeah?"

There was no response.

"Stella, are you there? Stella, are you okay??"

"I'm wiping, have bloody patience!" said Stella, taking another drag of her cigarette. "It's not so easy for girls, is it? It's tricky! You've got to—"

"Stella, I don't need to know all the details!" Frank felt the contents of his stomach rise to his oesophagus, and his diaphragm spasm. "Stella, we'll be home soon, alright? Leave the old bloke alone... do not hurt him!"

Frank hung up the phone, put his hands on his hips, and looked up into the sky. He looked very much like a superhero, albeit an old, very tired, and gravely ill superhero.

"Stan, I can't believe I'm saying this, but we're going to have to go home and sort this mess out," he said.

Stan looked crestfallen. "I know you're right, of course. But the race is tomorrow!" he said, devastated.

"I know, pal, I know, but there's nothing else we can do. There's simply nothing for it."

Fortunately for Frank and Stan, everyone was travelling to the Island rather than away from it, and they were able to get the first flight out in the morning

"I'm gutted," said Stan as the plane left the tarmac at Ronaldsway Airport. "Gutted."

"I know," said Frank. "And me as well. But we can still listen to it on the radio?" he added, trying to sound positive, though it was hard to pierce the pervading gloom. "Anyway, it was nice of Henk to invite us back in. Though I can't say I slept much last night. I'm devastated that we're not going to see the race, but the prospect that we may have been taken for a couple of chumps is really upsetting me even more. We've given Lee every opportunity to rebuild his life, to make a fresh start. He could have made a massive impact on other people's lives."

"As you said, Frank, it might be totally innocent," Stan offered.

"That's what I'd been trying to convince myself of all night long. But why would he go missing with the safe key? I hate to face up to facts, but I think we've been done over. Look, if we have been ripped off, can we keep it to ourselves? I'm going to put the money back into the charity account."

"We're going to put it back, you mean," said Stan. "I trusted Lee as much as you did, so don't think for a minute you're footing the bill on your own!"

"Cheers, mate," said Frank.

"Should we call the police?" asked Stan. "Y'know... if?"

"I've been thinking about that," replied Frank. "And I don't want to see the guy locked up. But I don't think we have much of a choice. If we don't get them involved, and people did find out, they might think we were in some way involved, or even worse, that we've tried to rip off the charity. I don't like it, but I think we'll have to."

Stan was presently staring at Frank rather intently.

"What is it?" said Frank. "What're you looking at me like that for?"

"Frank, are you okay?" said Stan, and Frank could tell from Stan's face that he was being quite serious. "Honestly, you look washed out. I think you should go to see the doctor once we've landed."

Frank's first reaction was to resist, but he did indeed feel washed out, and, if he looked it as well, he knew Stan's concern was well-placed. "Okay, mate," he said. "I will. And I'll even let you drive me!"

Two men wearing black overalls and motorcycle helmets entered the offices of Frank 'n' Stan's Taxis. This wasn't particularly unusual, in itself, as they had a courier delivery contract and they'd often have riders coming and going to the office each day.

Stella didn't even raise her head when the bell hung over the door chimed gently. She was engrossed in the *Times'* crossword puzzle and had a pen poised in one hand and a cigarette in the other.

"Give me the fucking money!" shouted one of the men, now stood in front of the desk.

Stella didn't flinch. "Seven across. Name of the theatre where Lincoln was assassinated," she said. She took the pen and began foraging in her ear with it.

"Money!" the man repeated, more aggressively.

Stella slowly looked up. "No, dickhead," she said, evenly. "It begins with an *eff.* As in, *eff* you, yeah?"

The two men turned to face each other, and for a moment it looked like they might disappear as quickly as they'd arrived.

"Give me the money! Now!" shouted the other man, stepping forward and taking a miniature cricket bat from inside his jacket. It was made for kids, obviously, or as a tourist souvenir, though it still looked of quite sturdy construction.

Stella was both unamused and unconcerned. "Bloody cricketers!" she cursed. "It's always the bloody cricketers, innit??"

"What?" said one of the intruders.

"That doesn't even—?" said the other.

And, then, ignoring them, "Now. You lot," Stella said, taking a long drag off her cigarette. "I can tell from the accents you're not from around these parts, so I feel obliged to educate you. See, in this country, taxi offices tend not to have a lot of cash hanging about. Think about it, yeah? When have you ever gone to a taxi office and paid the person behind the counter? You don't. You pay the taxi, don't you? Now, either you're very stupid, the pair of you, or you've mistaken me for the post office — which *does* have cash, and is down the street, just there."

She pointed in the direction of the post office, helpfully.

The two men looked at each, their expressions unreadable as their tinted visors were both down, and then back at Stella.

"If you both piss off now, right now, I'll extend you the courtesy of not telling them you're on the way, I promise."

Stella reached under the counter and calmly produced a bat of her own, revealing a rather large — and full-sized — American Louisville Slugger® baseball bat.

She went to casually rest it on her shoulder, but, as she began to do so, the man with the mini cricket bat in hand leant forward and swung, catching Stella on the side of the temple before she even knew what had happened.

She collapsed, with blood already pouring from her head before she hit the floor.

"We're not joking!" the man screamed. He walked behind the counter and grabbed Stella by the hair, pulling her upright — which was no mean feat. He marched her into the back office, and threw her against the desk.

"Open the fucking safe, or I'll open your fucking skull with this bat!" the man said. "And don't even think I won't! You've got one more chance!" the man shouted.

Stella was concussed; she could hardly stand, and struggled to string a sentence together. "I haven't got the key... I can't open the safe," she said. "Honestly."

"Last chance! Where is the key??" the man demanded.

"Are you daft?" Stella said, her anger getting the better, under the circumstance, of her common sense. The anger also focussed her speaking ability, concussion be damned.

"I just told you I don't have the key, didn't I? Your mate Lee has got the key, hasn't he? Perhaps you should have spoken to him before you bloody came in!"

Stella tried valiantly to remain on her feet, but her legs wobbled like a blancmange and gave out from under her.

The two men looked at each other, visor-to-visor, once again, apparently unsure what to do.

"Master criminals, you two," said Stella from the floor, the spirit not gone from her just yet.

Fortunately they ignored Stella for the moment, focussing their attention instead on locating the key. They ripped open the filing cabinet, throwing the contents all over the office. In frustration, they even upturned the desk. But the key was, of course, nowhere to be found as it was not there for the finding.

"Where is the key!" the one with the bat screamed, raising it above his head.

"Fuck you," said Stella, faintly but unmistakably.

The one looked at his accomplice, and then gripped the mini cricket bat with both hands, raising it over his head.

"I say! Put that down!" said a voice, rather unexpectedly, from the doorway. It was a voice full of confidence, and with an air of authority, fully expecting to be taken quite seriously.

"I said, put that down this instant! I shan't ask you chaps again!" He wasn't yelling. But the forcefulness of his voice gave the same effect.

Arthur had his neatly-pressed grey trousers pulled unnaturally high up his waist, covered by a knitted blue cardigan that was a smidgen too tight. He stood, chin up, and with one foot planted firmly behind him and the other leg bent at the knee and with the foot raised up, just slightly, heel off the floor. It looked very much like Arthur was stood at the ready, ready to spring into action at a moment's notice. The truth of the matter, as it happened, was that his altered stance merely stemmed from the onset of arthritis in his right knee, and he wished to simply take the weight off it. But the men assailing Stella needn't know that, of course.

"Look, old man. Turn around, leave quickly, and you won't get hurt."

Arthur picked up an umbrella that was resting underneath the wooden coat stand, making a show of tossing it up and then snatching hold of it mid-air, and then held it before him like fencing sabre.

"Gentlemen," he said assuredly. "I should rather say the same to you. Leave straightaway, this unpleasantness behind you, and you may yet make it through the day unscathed."

Arthur hoped he sounded convincing. He'd done a bit of acting in his younger days, and he was presently mustering all the reserves in that regard he could manage.

The two ruffians did not move. It was difficult to tell, their faces hidden as they were, if their reaction was one of fear, confusion, or contempt. Arthur, taking the initiative, advanced forth. He threw the umbrella in the air, tossing it round rather smartly, and grabbed it by its tip. Then, he swung the umbrella like Thor's hammer, Mjölnir, with the thick wooden handle landing a sharp strike on the nearest hooligan's helmet visor, resulting in quite a nice chip out of it and a spiderweb of cracks.

The helmeted man at the receiving end of Arthur's blow stumbled back, but regained his footing soon enough. The two would-be thieves seemed uncertain at this point what precisely to do next. Obviously they'd seen the James Bond films and such, so they were certainly well aware of the dangerous situation they'd suddenly found themselves in. Just as in China nearly everyone knows some sort of kung fu, similarly, in England, absolutely anyone could turn out to be a secret agent, even the most unassuming of gents — and especially the most unassuming of gents, actually. Who knew what this cardigan-wearing fellow's next move might be, or what he had in his hidden arsenal of gadgets and weapons? This umbrella, for instance, may not be an umbrella at all! It might, in point of fact, be a clever weapon of unknown strength or design.

"Hit the dickhead again," moaned Stella.

The one with the cracked visor wasn't waiting around for Arthur's next move. Taking no chances, he clenched his fist and punched Arthur hard in the stomach. Arthur sighed and crumpled to the floor like... well, like a thing that crumples easily to the floor.

"Attacking an old-age pensioner and a woman. Very classy, indeed," said Stella. "Your mums must be so proud!"

The man with the bat leaned toward Stella. "Wait, you're a woman?" he said in disbelief, even raising his visor up so he could get a better look.

He stood back up, lowering his visor again, and shook his head in defeat. "Shit, come on, let's get out of here," he said to his accomplice reluctantly. "These two have nothing we want."

Stella was in a bad way but didn't want to give them the satisfaction of knowing it. She waited for a moment till they'd left the building before dragging herself over to Arthur.

"Nice work old-timer, thank you. Are you okay? You almost had them fooled."

Arthur raised his forefinger, signalling he needed a moment, as he struggled to catch his breath, and refill the lungs that'd gotten the wind knocked out of them.

"I almost had myself fooled," Arthur said, able to speak again. And, then, "Who were they?" he asked, once he'd composed himself.

"That was your friend Lee, I expect, or at least some of his mates," replied Stella, trying to stem the flow of blood down her face, and dabbing at her temple with a large handkerchief she'd mysteriously produced from the depths of her bosom like a rabbit from a magician's hat.

"What should we do now?" asked Arthur.

"At times like this, I find it's always good to have a fag and a think. Do you want one?" she offered, reaching into her pocket.

"A fag or a think?" Arthur asked, confused.

"Yes," replied Stella.

Arthur shrugged his shoulders. "Sure," he said, ready to accept either.

"Didn't think I was a woman, did he?" Stella said to herself, lighting her fag. "I'm ALL woman!" she shouted out, as if the intruders could still hear her. "They don't know what they're bloody missing out on!"

chapter twenty-one

What the hell is going on here?" asked Stan. They pulled up to the taxi office and were greeted by several police cars and an ambulance, all with blue lights flashing.

"That's far enough," said a young constable, raising his arm to block their way.

"But that's our office. I'm Frank and he's Stan, as it says above the door."

The constable relented and escorted them into the office, after clearing it with his sergeant.

Stella was sat on the desk being tended to by a paramedic.

"Can you put your cigarette down for a moment?" asked the paramedic. "It's making it difficult to get neat stitches into the wound."

"Shit, Stella, are you okay? What the hell's happened here?? Did *he* do this to you???" asked Stan in a panic.

"Don't worry about that, love. If it leaves a scar, it'll match the one on the other side," replied Stella to the paramedic, taking a long drag. And, then, to Frank and Stan, "Ah, look what's washed ashore. Tweedledee and Tweedledum, The Bellend Boys, have finally decided to grace us with their presence. And did *who* do this to me? Two blokes tried to rob us, and I got hit with a bloody cricket bat across the head. Bloody cricketers!"

"What?" said Stan. "That doesn't even—?"

"I know, right? Why use a bloody mini bat when you could've used a full-sized one? It dun't make no sense!"

"No, that's not what—" Stan began.

"And if it wasn't for Grandad over there," Stella carried on, undaunted. "It could have been a lot worse."

"We need to get him to hospital," said the other paramedic, in reference to Arthur. "He's been struck pretty hard and I'm worried about internal bleeding."

"I've not finished with this one yet," replied the first.

"Don't you worry about that," Stella assured her. "I'll put the last couple of stitches in myself. I've always fancied myself the crafty type. You pair look after the old boy. He's who needs it most."

"Was it Lee?" asked Frank, after taking all this in. "Did he do this, Stella?"

Stella shrugged her shoulders. "They had helmets on, so I'm not sure. I'm fairly certain he wasn't one of them. But likely his mates, I expect — it's too much a coincidence that he turns up, knows there's a load of cash in the safe, and next thing we're being held up by armed robbers demanding the key to open it. Oh, and nobody has seen him since. Lee, that is."

Stan placed his hand on his forehead. From the look on his face, he was having trouble making sense of it. "I don't understand this, though. Stella, you said Lee had the key?"

Stella nodded.

"But why would the robbers need the key, then? If it was Lee that's done this, he already had the key?"

"Do I look like Hercule Poirot?" asked Stella. "Perhaps they'd arranged to meet up, or they thought the key was here? Who knows? Criminals aren't generally the cleverest of people. If they were, then they wouldn't be criminals in the first place. Whatever way you look at this, Lee arrived on the scene and we're getting robbed five minutes later and the bastard is now nowhere to be seen. If it looks like a duck, walks like a duck, and talks like a duck... it's a bloody duck, I says."

"Lovely day for it," Frank said weakly, and out of his head. "Good for the ducks."

"Frank?" said Stan.

"We need the rain," Frank said to no one in particular.

"Frank!" said Stan, rushing over to him. "Somebody give me a hand here!" he shouted to the police officer by the door. "Frank!"

Frank was still upright, just barely, but his eyes were rolling in his head. Beads of sweat covered his forehead.

"Help me!" shouted Stan as Frank fell forwards.

Fortunately, a second ambulance had arrived, believing there to be multiple casualties from the robbery, and Frank was soon to be accompanying Arthur in hospital.

Stan joined Stella and sat on the desk. "I'm sorry about all this, Stella. Are you feeling okay?"

"I'm fine," she said. "You needn't worry about me, I'm made of sterner stuff. Just a bit upset I didn't get a punch in, actually. You should've seen Arthur, Stan. He was bloody brilliant. I hate to admit it, but the old tosser may have just saved my life."

"You can punch me if you like," Stan offered.

"I may take you up on that later," said Stella. "Frank looks like shit, by the way. Was it the lighting in here or was his skin actually grey?"

"I think he's been doing too much. But honestly, Stella, he's had the best time of his life. I knew I should have told him to take it easy, but seeing the look on his face I knew he wouldn't have listened to me. Stella, he'll kill me for telling anyone, but he's refused any treatment."

"Tosspot," remarked Stella, though with very nearly a hint of affection.

"Why don't you get Susie in to cover and you get yourself home?" Stan offered. "We don't want our Stella keeling over as well. What would we do without you?"

"What, indeed?" Stella grunted. "True talent around here is rare as rocking horse shit. But, naw, I'm not going anywhere. You can't get rid of me that easily, and it'll take more than a couple of muppets wielding a glorified cocktail stick to send me packing. Besides, I want to be here in case those wazzacks come back, so's I can get a punch in next time!"

"That's the spirit," said Stan. "Look, I'll phone Molly and head down to the hospital. Tell the police that if they should need me, I'll pop in on the way back or they can call me. And that goes for you as well, alright?"

"Whatever," replied Stella, in her inimitable fashion.

Stan chuckled and turned to leave.

"Stan," said Stella just as he'd put his hand on the door. "Do us a favour and look in on the old boy, Arthur, yeah? He really did stop me getting another clump across the head. I don't think he's got anyone, and his only friend, Lee, has buggered off."

"I will, Stella. And promise you won't be a hero?"

"Get out of here," said Stella, "before I change my mind and punch you right now!"

Stan sat with Molly in the hospital waiting room for most of the afternoon. He kept his promise and looked in on Arthur, but the staff couldn't give him too much information as he wasn't family. He'd picked up an overnight bag for Frank, and he brought a spare pair of pyjamas and a toothbrush in for Arthur. They did tell him that they didn't think it was internal bleeding, in Arthur's case, but they were going to keep him under observation for a day or two.

Stan agonised about saying something to Molly about Frank's stubbornness. He didn't want to upset her any further at a time like this. On the other hand, he knew that if anyone could get through to Frank, it was her.

"You... know about the treatment?" he asked.

Molly held her head in her hands. "Yes," she said, her voice breaking. "Stan, I don't know what to do. My dad... I love him, Stan. I love him very much."

"He knows that, Molly," said Stan, putting his arm around her shoulders. "He loves you, a great deal, also." They'd been there for hours, and with Molly's mother being overseas, especially, he wanted to be by her side.

Every time the waiting room door opened, Stan's heart skipped a beat. It opened again, and they both looked up.

"Molly?" asked a young doctor who looked barely old enough to shave.

"Yes?" she replied, tentatively.

"You can come in and see your father now if you'd like."

"How is he?" she asked. "Is he awake?"

"Molly," the doctor said gently. "As you know, your father has underlying health issues. His immune system is very weak, and he's had a bit of a turn. It looks like he's just been doing a bit too much lately, a bit more than he should under the circumstances."

Stan bowed his head in guilt.

"Family?" the doctor asked, in reference to Stan.

"He's family," Molly said, rubbing his arm affectionately.

"Right, you can go in as well," said the doctor.

Frank was sat virtually upright, what with the volume of pillows he had stuffed behind him.

"No grapes?" he asked as they walked in the room.

Molly sobbed as she sat beside him and placed her head onto his chest. "You scared us," she said, trying to catch her breath. "The doctor thinks you've been doing too much!"

"What do they know?" said Frank, "I'm feeling fine now, right as rain. I think the news about Lee, and seeing Stella and the old boy out of sorts just got to me, is all."

"Yes, I'm sure that's all it was," Stan said, rolling his eyes.

"How is he, Stan?" asked Frank.

"Arthur? He's fine, I dropped him a pair of your pyjamas to borrow. I'm not really sure what to do, actually. There's nobody I can phone for him. According to Stella, if it wasn't for him, things could've been a whole lot worse."

"Who's this Arthur?" Molly asked.

"We don't really know too much about him quite yet," Stan explained, "But he—"

"Nevermind about that!" interjected Frank. "The race! While I've been laid up here, I've had no news!"

"Ah! Well!" said Stan. "As a matter of fact—"

"Out with it!" shouted Frank.

A nurse poked her head in. "Is everything all right in here? Shall I call the doctor?"

"We're okay," Molly assured her. "He's just a little excitable. This is normal for him."

The nurse padded off.

"I listened to the end of the race!" said Stan in a loud whisper. "They turned the radio in the waiting room on for us."

"And?" asked Frank, coming to attention.

"One-oh-four-point-six-one-three, fastest lap, and they finished eighteenth overall," said Stan, like a proud dad at parents' evening.

"That's bloody amazing news. Did you speak to Dave?"

"No, I sent him a text. I've not told him that you're in here. I thought we'd give him a ring tomorrow."

"I wish we'd have been there to see that," said Frank. "Molly, you have to come with us next year. It's the most unbelievable event you'll ever see, and me and Stan had our name on a sidecar!"

"I know, Stan showed me a picture," Molly said, smiling to hear him planning about the future. "Dad," she said. "Dad, I just wanted to say, I love you very, very much."

"Well of course you do," said Frank, stroking her back. "Of course you do. What's not to love?"

214

Molly remained curled into her dad like a cat, warm and cosy.

"And on that note," said Stan, rolling his eyes again, "I'll get us some coffee. Leave you two alone for a bit."

"Stan, before you go," said Frank. "There's something I wanted to tell you both."

Stan took a step closer and must have appeared concerned. "It's good news, Stan, don't worry," Frank reassured him. "I've spoken to the doctor, you know, about the treatment. I don't know how he does it, but he was able to speak to me like, well, a friend, rather than a doctor. I understood what he was saying to me and I've decided that I'm going to start the treatment, as soon as possible. I know the odds aren't stacked in my favour, but I want to try everything that I can."

"You'll beat this, Frank," Stan said, a wave of relief washing over him. "You're a stubborn bugger. And if anyone can do it, *you* can."

Stan waited in line at the coffee shop in the foyer, brushing a tear away from his cheek that had somehow mysteriously got there. Such was the extent of the smile on his face that perfect strangers were smiling back at him. Frank's announcement had been a huge relief, of course. The knots in his stomach had disappeared, and the pain in his lower back as well. It was amazing what stress could do. He'd blocked the thought of Frank's illness out as much as could, but the prospect of losing his friend was still always there.

Stan's mind drifted to thoughts of Dave and Monty. He was proud of them, proud of what they'd accomplished, and was happy to have been a part of it.

There must have been over a hundred people nearby, milling about, with the accompanying murmur of voices. One voice in particular, though, made Stan's ears prick up, clear above all the others: a familiar lilting Irish accent.

He slowly turned, taking a side-step, and cocked his head for a better listen.

"That's bloody Lee," he said under his breath.

The queue in front of Stan had moved forward without him, and a woman behind him coughed, and then coughed again.

"Sorry, you go on," said Stan, stepping out of line.

He couldn't be one-hundred percent certain, but he caught sight of what he was fairly sure was Lee, walking off with a rather attractive woman with long, blonde hair.

Stan took off in pursuit, and reached for his phone. "Shit!" he said, realising that in all the rush to get to hospital he'd left his phone in the car.

Stan had seen plenty of surveillance scenes in the movies and so knew the drill, and he stayed back, kept out of sight. With the stealth of a very stealthy person, he'd been able to confirm that it was indeed Lee he'd set his sights on, and had thoughts of running up and planting one directly on his chin.

"Shit, Arthur," said Stan, as the lift doors closed, with Lee and his blonde companion — accomplice? new target? — behind them.

Stan rushed up and pressed the lift button impatiently, again and again, as thoughts of shouting out for security ran through his mind. The only reason that Lee would be there was... to see Arthur? It must've been. Did he think Arthur had the safe key? Or, perhaps he was angry that Arthur had foiled his robbery, and he was there for revenge?

Stan felt sick, and for someone who never ran, he was in full sprint through the hospital corridor once off the lift.

Stan arrived at Arthur's room, but the door was ajar, and the room was empty. His heart sank when he saw the freshly made bed, ready for the next occupant.

A nurse was walking by, escorting an elderly patient. Stan accosted her.

"Excuse me, Miss. Do you know where the chap who was in this room went?"

"Are you family?" she asked.

"Yes," said Stan, lying for the greater good.

"He's been moved onto the main ward," she said, pointing to where she'd just come from.

There were six beds on the ward, and, once there, Stan scanned the room.

"Lee, you piece of shit!" shouted Stan.

"Stan, how are you?" said Lee, smiling, surprised by Stan's form of address but having to assume it was nothing more than some friendly piss-taking.

... One second before Stan punched him square on the bridge of the nose.

Stan had never punched anyone in his life, and, for his debut effort, he certainly made impressive contact.

"What the fucking fuck?" said Lee, holding onto his face. "What the hell was that for?"

"What the hell are you doing here, and what have you done with all the cash? I see you've managed to hook up with some pretty tart already. Did you tell her you were some rich bigshot, with all of your stolen money?"

"Keep the noise down!" said the furious-looking matron. "Do I need to call security??"

"No, it's fine," said Lee, wiping the blood from his nose. "Stan, have you gone completely mad?" asked Lee. "What on earth are you on about??"

"As if you didn't know," said Stan. "And where's your tart gone?"

Lee reached for the curtain covering the end bed. Once pulled back, there was the pretty tart, leaning over Arthur, holding him in her arms.

"Stan," said Lee. "The pretty tart is Arthur's daughter. Did Stella not get in touch with you?"

The pretty tart looked over at them for a moment.

"I'm not a tart," she said.

"Arthur, are you okay in there?" asked Stan, suspiciously.

Arthur smiled at Stan. "I'm brilliant, thank you. The best I've ever been, in fact. I've got my beautiful, lovely daughter back!" he said. "I've got my wonderful daughter back. Wait, hang on... why are you calling my daughter a tart?" he said.

"A pretty tart," Arthur's daughter corrected.

"I, uh... oh, dear," said Stan.

Lee walked towards Stan with his hands held up, palms out, in submission. "You're not going to hit me again, I hope?"

Stan, for his part, said nothing at this point, but looked a mixture of baffled and ashamed.

"I told Arthur to meet at the taxi office as I had a surprise for him," Lee began. "You now know what that surprise was," he explained.

"Hiya," said Arthur's daughter with a cheery wave.

"But when we arrived," Lee continued, "Stella told us what had happened. Funnily enough, she also tried to punch me. Look, Stan, I didn't try and steal anything, I can promise you."

"But what about the key?" Stan protested weakly. "Stella said you had the key to put the charity cash in?"

"I did put the cash in the safe. I then gave the key back to Stella. She was on the phone, and I dropped it in her handbag. She can't have been paying attention, because when we looked just now, it was there. Where it's always been, the whole time."

"And the cash..."

"Is there! Where it's always been, the whole time! Don't worry. Stella said she was going to call you and tell you we were on the way."

"Ah," said Stan. "I left my phone in the car. So there's that."

Stan was feeling very guilty now about the blackening forming on Lee's eyes. He coughed uncomfortably. "So, em... where did you find Arthur's daughter?"

"The pretty tart?" said Arthur's daughter, smiling.

"Yes, well, sorry about—" Stan began.

"At least you were half right," said Arthur, and they all had a laugh, and Stan didn't feel quite such an ass as he just had a moment ago.

"She wasn't that hard to find," said Lee, answering Stan's question. "The problem for Arthur was that he never had social media! It took me less than half an hour to find her on Facebook. And she thought her dad hadn't wanted anything to do with her! Can you imagine?"

Stan took a moment to absorb the information. "Lee, I'm sorry! Sorry for thinking you'd taken the money, and sorry for punching you."

Lee shrugged. "It wasn't the first time I've been punched, believe me," he said, smirking.

"Was it a good punch, by the way?" asked Stan. "Could you tell it was my first time, or—?"

"It was very good, Mr Balboa. Or can I call you Rocky?" said Lee.

"Rocky is fine," said Stan, looking at the floor, smiling.

"If I ever need to hire any muscle, you'd be my first choice," Lee assured him. "Closely followed by Stella."

"Ta, for that. Look, sorry again. I need to get back to Frank. I left him twenty minutes ago, to get him coffee. We'll catch up tomorrow, have a chat about the charity and the next steps? Great job reuniting them, Lee, fantastic work."

Stan waved at Arthur and his daughter, and pretended to shadowbox with Lee on his way out.

He stopped suddenly as if he'd walked right into the door — even though it was wide open.

"Hang on. If you didn't try and rob the money, then who did? And how did they know the money was in the safe in the first place? I need to get that cash out of the safe and then I think I need to phone the police, because if everyone thinks it was you, then nobody's looking for the actual criminals. Shit, they're still out there — what if they come back again?"

chapter twenty-two

"You look happy, Stella?" said Stan.

With her headset on, she hadn't heard him coming and threw her mobile phone hastily into her drawer.

"Don't sneak up on people!" she shouted.

"Okay, calm down. What were you up to?" asked Stan, clearly fishing.

"And that's your business, how?" she said.

"It's none of my business. I was just pleased to see you pleased, is all."

"Bloody Molly's blabbed, hasn't she?"

Stan held his hands out to protest his innocence. "A little bit, yes, but she's just happy for you. Would you show me? I've often wondered how this internet dating thing worked."

Stella reluctantly pulled her phone out the drawer. "If you're teasing me, Stan, the only dating site you'll need is Eunuchs-dot-com because I'll rip your testicles off!"

"No, I'm being serious," replied Stan, subconsciously using his hands to cover his groin.

Stella logged onto the app with Stan stood over her shoulder. "You create a profile on here and people, if they like you, get in touch," she explained. "Simples!"

"It's all a bit mercenary, isn't it? What about the good old days of walking up to someone in a bar and buying them a drink? Wait, who's she?" said Stan, pointing at the profile picture.

"That's my profile picture," replied Stella.

"But, that's not you?" he said, moving closer. He strained his eyes. "Is that not Brigitte Nielsen?"

"I don't know, I found it on the internet."

"Stella, she's quite famous. She was married to Rocky."

Stella rolled her eyes. "His wife was Adrian, dickhead."

"No, I mean in real life," said Stan. "Bloody hell, Stella, you can actually see Sylvester Stallone behind her in that picture."

She shrugged her shoulders. "Dun't matter, I've already had a few people getting in touch."

"But what do you do when they show up and see...?"

"See what?" she said, storm clouds forming over her head.

"See that you're not Ivan Drago's wife," Stan said.

"Who?" said Stella. "I thought you said she was married to Rocky?"

"Wait..." said Stan. Now he was getting himself confused.

"Now you're talking about chemical engineers," Stella groused.

Now Stan was lost. "Chemical—?"

"Ivan Drago!" said Stella. "He's got a master's in chemical engineering in real life! Don't you know anything?"

"Apparently, I..." Stan shook his head to clear his mind. "Okay, forget about all that. Anyway, I think I'll just go back to the traditional approach of actually speaking to people. Look, Frank's on his way in so don't be getting his blood pressure up. I've got a little surprise for him, so if you've got any problems with it, wait till he's gone and you can take it up with me."

Stella was about to erupt into a rant when Stan — rather bravely — placed a solitary finger over her mouth.

"Stella," he said. "You've held things together around here, and will probably need to do a bit more over the next few months. I've been speaking with Frank, and we're going to increase your salary by a thousand pounds a month as our way of saying thank-you."

Stella frowned. "That's all I'm worth, a crappy thousand pounds a month for all the shit I put up with from you two idiots?"

Stan looked hurt, before she stood and put her arms around him.

"I'm only kidding, you big orange-faced idiot," she said, planting a kiss in the middle of his forehead. "And, for what it's worth, I've quite enjoyed having Lee and Arthur in the office. But don't tell them that, I want to maintain a certain level of healthy fear, understood?"

"I think so, Brigitte. Mum's the word, you can count on me," Frank told her. "Oh, here we go. Frank's back."

It'd been difficult to keep Frank away from the office, as for those that worked there, it was more of a social club than a place of work. Frank had been in hospital for three days, more to keep him under observation than anything else. But, aside from the underlying health issues, he was looking good.

"Frank, Frank, Frank," said Stan, giving his friend a warm embrace.

"You two look suspiciously suspicious," said Frank, eying them warily.

"Nonsense, we're just happy to be in work, isn't that so, Stella? We were just reminiscing about our favourite Rocky film. You don't look too happy to be back?"

"I'm fine. I've just been down the police station."

"What for, they didn't phone me?" said Stan, slightly offended.

"It wasn't about the robbery here," replied Frank. "Well, not technically."

"Have they given you too much medication?" asked Stella.

Frank took his jacket off. "Stella, any chance of a coffee?"

"I don't see why not. Stan? I'll take one as well, thanks."

Stan began to open his mouth but Stella cut him short. "I'm only joking," she said. "Stan, would you like one?"

Stan waited for the other shoe to drop, but it never did. "I'd love one, Stella, thanks."

"She actually is getting us coffee?" Frank asked, after Stella had left the room. "I never thought—"

"Don't you dare tell her I said this, but I think she's happy to see you back," Stan said, then looked at Frank expectantly. "Anyway. You were saying?"

"Yes," continued Frank. "The police called me this morning. They had a phone call last night about suspicious behaviour by the house. Having nosey bastards for neighbours seems to have paid off for once. Fortunately, Helen is still away at her sister's, but they caught someone still hanging around."

"Shit, did they get anything?" asked Stan.

"Well, that was the peculiar thing, wasn't it? He'd been in the house, all right. Left everything of value, oddly enough. Found only one thing on him."

Frank paused there, for dramatic effect, much to the annoyance of Stan and Stella.

"Yes? And...??" shouted Stan. "So what did they find on him??"

Frank savoured the moment, keeping them in suspense just a bit longer, before saying...

"He had taken a bunch of keys."

"That's it?" asked Stella. "Do they know who it was?"

Frank nodded. "It was Boris, as it turned out. The one Helen kicked into touch the other week."

"What? Why would he break in to get keys? Did he not move in with her?" asked Stan.

"He didn't move in, but she changed all of the locks as he had a key."

"Right, I'm getting confused now," said Stan. "So he broke in to steal the keys for the new lock?"

Frank shook his head. "No, that's what the police thought, at first. They found his friend sat waiting in a car, around the corner. They arrested him and searched the car, and guess what they found?"

"My will to live??" said Stella.

"No! They found two black crash helmets, one with a crack in the visor thanks to our resident pit bull, Stella."

Stella had a face like thunder.

"Boris and his mate are the ones that robbed us?"

"Apparently so. After Helen kicked him out, he had no money — she'd been funding his lifestyle. Well, I suppose I was, by default. Anyway, the police checked his mobile and found that he'd tried to phone me dozens of times when we were in the Isle of Man. He must have seen our TV interview, and saw Lee as the perfect scapegoat for their robbery attempt. And it very nearly worked perfectly."

"Ah," said Stan. "And when the key wasn't here at the office, they assumed that you'd have a spare at the house?"

"Exactly," said Frank. "And, unfortunately for them, they were correct, I did have a key... BUT, I always kept it separate in case Helen decided to go on a shopping spree or get her boobs upgraded. So bad luck for them. Anyway, it seems like Boris and his friend are also wanted in their motherland and have a very eager detective travelling over, just waiting for the chance to ask them a few questions. Those two are going to jail for a very, very long time."

"I'm not really sure how to top that, Frank, if I'm being honest, but, I have a surprise for you." Said Stan.

"Okay," said Frank slowly. "What's that?"

"What day is tomorrow?" Stan asked.

"Is it a trick question? It's Friday, surely?" replied Frank.

Stan waved his hand in front of him in a circular motion, trying to draw greater details out of him, but his efforts were fruitless.

"What happens tomorrow in the Isle of Man?" he said, giving him a hint.

Frank looked confused. "Senior Race day?"

"Senior Race day. That's correct, my fine old friend. And we'll be cheering Dave and Monty on in the sidecar race."

Frank's face lit up. "Seriously??"

"Seriously!" said Stan. "I spoke with Henk and it's all sorted."

Frank's smile turned to confusion and consternation.

"Stan, I've experienced your travel plans first-hand, and if it was a challenge to get to the Isle of Man in practice week, what hope have we got for Senior Race day?"

"Helicopter?" said Stella, nonchalantly.

Stan scowled at her. "Stella! You've ruined my bloody surprise!"

"You've not got us a helicopter?" said Frank, eyes wide like a child at Crimbo.

"I bloody well have, Frank. Molly spoke with your doctor and he's fine with it. We leave at tea-time in our very own helicopter!"

"Oh, Stanley," said Frank. "Stanley, Stanley. This is another really fine mess you've got us into. You little beauty!!"

If the Island was glorious at ground level, it was captivating from the air. Fortunately, the pilot was a TT enthusiast and frequent flyer to the Isle of Man. He took them on a gentle detour and followed the TT course to give them a sense of perspective from their unique vantage point. They'd set off early as the sidecar race was the first on the schedule for the day's racing. Senior Race day was the culmination of the fortnight, with the festival closing, at the very end, with the Blue Riband event: the gruelling six-lap Senior TT for the solo machines.

The contrast between the lush, tree-covered roads at sea level, and the rolling green, barren landscape of the mountain section was apparent. Frank and Stan absorbed the landscape in wonderment, and, happily, the weather had played its part with brilliant blue skies and vibrant sunshine glistening off the still Irish Sea as they landed at Ronaldsway Airport in the south of the Island.

"You need to put these on," said Stan, handing Frank a set of rather unattractive blue overalls.

Frank stared blankly.

"We've got passes to watch the races from the pit area and we need to wear these for safety. Dave was eager to sign us up for his pit crew, but I didn't think we were cut out to fill our *own* petrol tanks, let alone *his* in the middle of the race."

"That's going to be amazing!" said Frank. "I'm lactating like Pavlov's dog!"

"Don't you mean saliva–?" Stan replied, but stopped short. "You know what, it doesn't matter. Lactating like Pavlov's dog it is, then," said Stan giddily, unwilling to break the spell.

The journey from the airport took a leisurely twenty minutes, but the traffic was amplified by those taking advantage of the roads before they closed for most of the day. As they approached the Quarterbridge roundabout, the sight was breathtaking.

"Holy shit!" said Stan. "That's absolutely crazy!"

"Fooking mental!" Frank agreed, mesmerised.

Every inch of pavement outside the pub was crammed with spectators soaking up the morning sunshine. The field opposite where the temporary campsite was erected was peppered with anxious heads peering over the stone wall, and as the lads progressed through the junction they saw hundreds more sat on a grass bank which formed a natural earthen seating area. The familiar dulcet tones of Chris Kinley filled the atmosphere once again, and the sound waves held in the air were comforting and welcoming, wrapping around Frank and Stan like a warm blanket on a cold evening.

They knew Dave and Monty would be otherwise occupied, but hoped a quick detour would give them the opportunity to wish them well.

For a man who was about to go racing around the TT course, Dave was remarkably relaxed as he sat in what might be best described as the Lotus position... assuming you viewed him a certain special way. It was like one of those picture books with the hidden images that can only be seen if you look at them without really looking at them, and it's only then that the image forms, but if you look straight at it then it's gone.

"Monty, good luck, mate!" whispered Stan. "I wanted to say hello to Dave, but I think he's meditating... or something."

"No," said Monty. "The fat bastard has been eating cheeseburgers all week. He's trying to stretch the leather so he can get fasten the—"

"Ah, Stan," said Dave. "Give us a hand, will you? Get yourself over here and help me with this zip, yeah?"

Dave remained on the floor with his shoulders arched forward, with Stan standing over him, crotch-to-face, straddling him with legs on either side.

The TV coverage team were moving around the paddock to try and convey the electricity for those watching the highlights from home. They panned the camera onto Stan's back, where his hands were hidden in front as he grasped Dave's zip. "It's coming," said Stan. "I'm almost there!" Dave's head was inches from Stan's waist, and, though mostly obscured by the camera, could nevertheless be made out quite clearly bobbing like a Nodding Donkey in a Texas oilfield each time Stan pulled at the zip.

"Of all the pre-race rituals we've witnessed," said the commentator. "That's certainly the most, ahem... friendly... we've seen. No judgement. Good luck, guys!"

Later, with Dave's costume sorted, Frank and Stan felt like celebrities as they flashed their pit passes, allowing access to the starting grid. They stood on Glencrutchery Road — a few yards from the start line — as the earlier-numbered sidecars were wheeled out to their starting positions. It was still early, but the heat was radiating from the tarmac below.

"They must be bloody boiling in leather, sat on them bikes," said Frank, wiping the sweat from his face.

"That's got to be Chris Kinley," said Stan. "I feel like we know him already from listening to him."

"He's smaller than I thought," replied Frank.

Chris bobbed and weaved around the grid like a bantamweight boxer. He appeared from nowhere, thrusting his microphone into the faces of unsuspecting racers, before quickly moving on to the next. Frank and Stan followed, listening intently to a consummate professional, getting as close as they could.

Chris did a quick change direction, once again, but Frank and Stan didn't react in time and ploughed straight into the back of him.

"If you two don't stop following me, I'm going to stick this microphone right up your..."

"... and Dave Quirk, Number Forty-Two and a top local prospect," he said, on cue, back into the mic, remaining composed.

Frank and Stan retreated, offering Dave and Monty a wave of encouragement. "We sponsor them," said Stan, to anyone within earshot. "That's our name. On the side. Just there," he continued, beaming. People smiled and nodded, humouring the crazy person.

The sound of the klaxon, followed by an announcement from the clerk of the course, saw the road cleared, apart from the racers. In an instant, dozens of press, sponsors, and officials left the riders alone with their thoughts. The focus on the racers' faces was intense; it was difficult to comprehend how they felt moving toward the starting arch, waiting patiently for the green light and a tap on the shoulder from the official. For the first rider away, there was clear tarmac in front and three laps of the 37.73 miles of the course — which was, without question, the most challenging motorsport event on earth.

Frank and Stan were stood on the opposite side of fuelling stations on pit lane as the race began. Nearly on top of them now, as they were, the sound of the screaming engines was both deafening and exhilarating, and the vibrations reverberated through every bone in their bodies.

"Here's Dave!" shouted Frank. "Go on, son!" they both shouted, waving their fists. They didn't realise it, but they were holding onto each other's arms like a young couple at a horror movie.

As soon as the visual stimulation of the bikes leaving was complete, a few minutes later and the first bikes away were approaching Glen Helen.

In race week, the two timing points also became commentary positions on Radio TT, with Dave Christian at Glen Helen and the stalwart of the TT, the legendary Roy Moore, at Ramsey Hairpin. They didn't have the time to announce all of the riders through, so spectators were also glued to the mobile app on their phones to monitor the progress of their favourites. The riders themselves had to rely on strategically-placed friends or associates holding out boards around the course to understand their current position. In a tight race, the position could change several times in a lap so information around the course was vital for those vying for a spot on the podium.

The front six riders on the opening lap were separated by only a smidgen over two seconds, which, considering the distance travelled, was remarkable. The commentary team around the course did a spectacular job bringing the race to life, and the enthusiasm over the radio waves maintained the proper tension.

"I'm buying a house over here," said Frank, matter-of-fact.

Stan gave him a look, unsure if he was being serious.

"I mean it," said Frank. "This is the most unbelievable place I've ever been to, and it's only twenty minutes away from home. Oh, and I'd like to put my holiday request in for two weeks leave, this time next year."

Stan smiled. "The thought had crossed my mind, also. About the house, that is. I expect we'll have to let Stella know we're both going to be off on holiday at this same time, next year."

The klaxon sounded to announce the imminent arrival of the first riders to complete their opening lap. Most had enough fuel onboard and so were unlikely to pull in, but the pit crew were like coiled springs, at the ready to refuel or make adjustments at a moment's notice should the need arise.

The grandstand, which had been relatively subdued for the last few minutes, was violated as three outfits went over the start line, inches apart. Frank and Stan felt punch-drunk as they watched in awe.

"They're going quick!" said Stan. And, then, looking at his phone, he added, "They're in fourteenth place!" He jumped on the spot, dancing a jig. "That's bloody amazing!"

"It must be those leathers being a bit too tight — maybe it's helped the wind resistance!" said Frank. "Hang on, here they come!"

Like a big fast boiled sweet, Dave and Monty hurtled past the grandstand and, with the goosebumps on Frank and Stan's skin, it felt like they'd fallen in a nettle bush.

"They're currently quicker than Harry McMullan!" shouted Stan. "Imagine they get their hundred-and-five-per-hour lap and beat that arsehole!"

"No way," said Frank. "They can't have done. No offence to Dave, but McMullan must have pulled over to make adjustments or something. Still... COME ON, DAVE!"

They waited impatiently for the mobile app to update and the timing to refresh.

"You know, Stan, I'm really pleased about Lee. I'm ashamed to admit that I'd written him off, and, from what he's said, that's what most people have done all his life."

"You're not alone, Frank. He's a good 'un. But with the information we had, what else were we supposed to think? I quite like the old boy as well, Arthur. Lee's eager to get him onboard to help out with the charity, and I think he should?"

"I totally agree," said Frank. "Plus, Arthur has done what many people have failed at, and made a friend out of Stella! I think this charity is going to grow quickly, and, without being morbid, in some ways I see it as a legacy. It's helped Lee and Arthur, and I can see this going national. It's really given me something to focus on."

"What I want right now," Stan said, "I want you to focus on us coming back here next year and staying in your new holiday home, and us watching Dave and Monty breaking a-hundred-and-ten miles an hour."

"I can't hardly argue with that," replied Frank.

Dave was taking advantage of every horsepower the bike gave him. She was running like a dream and the gearing and suspension — despite the lack of practice — were perfect. The conditions on the mountain section were faultless and as he slowed to negotiate the bend at the Creg-ny-Baa, about three miles from the start line, he knew it was going to be a quick lap, and Monty was playing his part as well — he'd been as reliable as the bike.

There was sufficient fuel in the tank to fly through the start line and onto his third and final lap without stopping. He kept his head tucked in and couldn't help but smile, glancing at the iconic scoreboard as he powered through the grandstand and into the sharp descent on Bray Hill.

He could usually relax into a race, but this was on a different level. The extra horsepower in the engine required even more intense concentration and his eyes were as wide as saucers. He'd negotiated Ballagarey with pinpoint precision on the previous two laps, but that didn't stop him holding his breath as he resisted every urge in his body that told him to slow down. The momentum he retained in the corner propelled along the stretch to Crosby, where he caught a fleeting glimpse of an outfit at the top of the road.

"McMullan," he said to himself.

He retained his composure and as much as he wanted to catch him up, he knew he had to ride his own race. Also, if he was coming up on McMullan on the road, he knew that McMullan'd had some sort of issue that'd slowed him down. Dave knew that if he were patient and maintained his pace, he'd have no problem in reeling them in.

Dave had visibly caught Tony Dearie and Harry McMullan on the run through Greeba Castle and Appledene, and he thought he'd be able to pass on the stretch coming up to the sharp right-hander at Ballacraine, but unfortunately the road ran out before he was able to safely overtake.

Dave dropped the bike down the gearbox and applied the brakes as he watched the line that Tony Dearie took, hoping to exploit the slightest error.

"Shit!" shouted Dave as the bike weaved for a moment as he entered the corner. He thought he'd lost control, and for a split-second he headed directly to the grass bank on the left-hand side. For a moment he thought perhaps the tyre had burst, but, luckily, this was not the case. He eased off the throttle, just enough, and wrestled with the steering, muscling the bike into a straight line once again. He glanced over his shoulder and caught sight of the sun glistening off an enormous oil slick trailing in his wake; he knew the leak was terminal. He raised his left hand to indicate to any outfit behind that he was slowing to pull over, but, as he did, noticed the trail of oil was stretched out in front of him as well.

"Bloody hell. It's Dearie that's leaking!" he said aloud.

Monty had raised his head when the bike slowed, but soon returned to his position when Dave pinned the throttle once again.

Dearie and McMullan were unaware of the oil leak, and pressed on with their bike running below optimum. Dave soon caught him on the winding section into Glen Helen and began to furiously wave to McMullan. As Dave pulled as close behind as he could, McMullan misread the gesture and, like the previous time, extended his arm and raised his middle finger in salute.

With the amount of oil that was flowing out Dearie and McMullan's bike, Dave knew that a few drops on the front wheel of his own would have catastrophic results. He pulled out from behind them and the oil trail, and he accelerated until he was alongside. The road was narrowing, and Dearie didn't expect an overtake in this position. Dearie turned his head for a moment, and, since he'd got his attention, Dave continued to motion with his hand.

They were travelling at about 135 mph. "Pull over, you knob!" Dave shouted, but there was no chance the other team could hear.

Fortunately, Tony was not as stupid as his passenger and eased off the throttle for a moment and lifted his head. Their speed dropped quickly, and, like Dave just before, Tony raised his hand to signal his intentions.

Before either of them were able to progress, Dave heard a sound like a cannon discharging and witnessed a cloud of black smoke erupt from Dearie's machine. At the fantastic rate of speed they were travelling, neither had time to react.

Dearie's bike smashed into Dave and Monty.

Monty was thrown from the bike as it flipped sideways, and he careered out of control through the air and onto the grass bank, his head just having missed an ornate stone wall.

Dave came to rest in the centre of the road and, by the grace of God, Tony Dearie's machine missed him — by only inches.

The marshals on duty responded immediately, and professionally. They ran towards the carnage with red flags being waved furiously to warn the other riders, and to bring the race to a halt.

Sidecar Number Forty-Two tumbled over and over in a trail of sparks, leaving gouges in the tarmac, coming, finally, to a sickening halt. It sat, upside down, with the wheels still spinning and petrol spilling onto the track.

Dave still lay on the road, and Monty on the grass shoulder. Neither of them were moving.

chapter twenty-three

Red Flag on track! Racing has been suspended due to a red flag on track! We'll bring you more information as soon as we have it...

Frank and Stan didn't need the radio to tell them what they could already see, the red flags waving. It was like a punch to the stomach.

"It's probably nothing. Maybe a sheep on the course, or something daft like that," said Stan, although the furrows on his forehead couldn't hide his concern.

The bikes nearest to the grandstand were instructed back via the return ramp, and although Frank knew Dave was miles away, he still watched every bike, willing it to be Dave.

The vibrant atmosphere had turned sombre, and the classic rock anthems on the radio failed to lift the spirits.

Minutes seemed like hours, as Stan and Frank stood in silence. They watched the faces of anybody who looked official, desperate for any indication, until finally the music was interrupted by the commentator:

An update on the red flag incident. We've had notification from Race Control that there has been an incident involving two bikes — Number Forty-Two, Quirk and Montgomery, and Number Eight, Dearie and McMullan. The riders have been flown to Nobles Hospital, but there is no update on their condition at this time. Race Control has confirmed the Sidecar Race will not be restarted, and all bikes are being escorted back to the grandstand by the travelling marshals.

The blood drained from their faces and Frank and Stan stood there, stunned.

"Shit," said Stan quietly, putting his hands to his face. "I don't know what we should do. Bloody hell, guys, please be okay."

Frank couldn't bring himself to even speak.

Frank and Stan delayed their return leg on the helicopter and took a taxi to the hospital. They waited for hours but as they weren't family the staff were unable to tell them anything. A flurry of visitors hurried through the waiting room, but as they were unsure if they were related to any of the riders, or simply visitors, Stan and Frank didn't want to upset anyone by interrupting.

Frank periodically checked the internet on his phone to see if there were any updates, but there was nothing.

"I'm worried," said Stan. "If everything was okay, they'd have surely said something by now?"

"I'm not sure there's too much we can do here," Frank replied, sighing. "Do we just head back home and see if there's any more information in the morning?"

Stan reflected for a few moments before answering. "I think you're right," he said. "We've been sat here for most of the day and we don't know anything. We could very well sit here all night and still not know anything. Perhaps we should leave our details with one of the nurses, and, if possible, pass our details over to one of their family, also."

Frank looked up and something caught his attention.

"Is that not Dave's brother Brian over there? The one who was helping him in the pits?" he asked.

Stan stared as much as he thought he could without appearing too obvious. "Yes! Yes, I think it is," he agreed. "Do you think we ought to go over and ask him?"

Frank stood and walked slowly towards the counter where the man he suspected was Brian was. He waited for a moment for a nurse to leave.

"Excuse me, I'm very sorry to bother you, but are you Dave's brother?"

Dave's brother nodded.

"Right, I'm Frank," Frank said. "My friend Stan and I have become friends with Dave and Monty. We don't live on the Island, and need to return home, and we wondered if you'd be kind enough to perhaps give us a phone and let us know how they are?"

Brian looked at Frank with suspicion for a moment, until there was a flicker of recollection. "You're the guys who helped them with the engine," he said. "The taxi owners?"

"Yes, that's us," said Frank. "We didn't know what else to do, so we've been waiting to see if anybody could give us any information. If you could call us, we'd be exceptionally grateful."

Brian took the piece of paper with the phone number that Frank handed him. "I'd be happy to, but I don't think we'll know anything today. I don't know anything about the other riders, mind you, but Dave is in a bad way."

"I'm sorry to hear that," said Frank, heart sinking. "We're really very fond of Dave and Monty. If you have the opportunity, will you tell them that we're thinking of them and praying for a speedy recovery?"

"Of course," said Brian. "If you don't mind, I really need to get back to the family."

"Cheers," said Frank.

The helicopter journey earlier in the day had been full of enthusiasm and hope, but as Stan and Frank took to the air at

Ronaldsway Airport for the journey home, there was a sense of despair.

The sun fell over the pretty coastal town of Peel in the West of the Island, cloaking it in a soft, golden glow, but Frank and Stan couldn't appreciate the beauty of it just now.

"This isn't how I wanted to leave the Island," said Stan. "I'd pictured us sharing a glass of champagne on the return trip, to toast Dave and Monty getting their hundred-and-five-mile-per-hour lap."

"They didn't finish the race," said Frank. "But at least they got the lap speed they were looking for — and then some. I hope Brian has been able to tell them that they got a-hundred-and-seven miles per hour on that last of theirs."

At work the next morning, Stella sent them home early. They didn't argue with her.

There was nothing on the news and nobody had phoned, and the lack of information was gnawing at them. They sat in Stan's kitchen and watched the footage they'd recorded on their phones with a great, but sad, fondness.

"Who's that?" asked Stan, as Frank's phone began to vibrate — indicating an incoming call. "It's a private number," he said, after seeing the number come up on Frank's screen.

Frank was both desperate to answer but reluctant to answer, knowing what might be at the other end.

"Hello," he said. His throat had constricted, his voice hoarse, and he could barely manage the word.

Stan turned away as he didn't want to misinterpret any of Frank's facial expressions. He listened intently.

"Yes, this is Frank," he said. "Brian, hi, how are you? Good news I—?"

There followed from Frank, interspersed with periods of silence, a series of grunts and short, one-word responses, which revealed to Stan nothing of discernible value.

"Okay, I see," said Frank, with an intonation which suggested that the conversation was coming to an end.

The suspense was driving Stan mad, and he turnt back around to look at Frank, anxious to glean anything he possibly could.

"Brian, it can't have been easy, and Stan and I both want to thank you for phoning, and we both send our very best wishes to you all," Frank concluded, ending the call.

Chris Kinley cleared his throat and brought the audience to order.

"I'd like to thank you all for attending this evening, on what is relatively short notice. As you all know, we're here because of the horrendous accident in the second sidecar race. We're honoured to be invited to Government House, in the presence of the Lieutenant Governor of The Isle of Man, and I'd like to bring his excellency onto the stage in a few moments...

"If we can take away anything from an awful incident, it's the spirit of true sportsmanship and selfless action embodied in our beloved sport, as evidenced and demonstrated so beautifully by David Quirk and Shaun 'Monty' Montgomery in this last race. The Spirit of TT Award is given to recognise those heroes who have demonstrated a contribution to the TT or a moment of excellence. This is ordinarily awarded on Senior Race Day, but in view of the moment of excellence we saw from outfit Number Forty-Two, the sponsors and organisation committee wanted to postpone the award until such time as it could be properly presented. Which brings us, of course, to today."

A pause was given, so that the crowd could show their appreciation.

"What I'd like to do now," Chris continued. "Is invite Harry McMullan onto the stage, if I may."

The crowd gave Harry a rapturous round of applause as he made his way onto the stage with the assistance of a pair of crutches. For a man who was usually brash, bordering on arrogant, he was humble now, with his head bowed.

"The Spirit of TT award has often passed me by, if I'm being honest with myself," McMullan said, speaking into the mic. "I mean, I know what it is, but previously I've not paid it any attention. Am I proud of that? No I'm not. I'm here to tell you, that no I'm not...

"Since the accident, where I've had first-class treatment at the hospital, I've had a lot of time to think about the people that give so much to make this event so special. Dave Quirk and Shaun Montgomery should be on this stage with me right now. They did something that, I'm embarrassed to admit, I'm not sure I could have or would have done myself...

"Those who know me will know I can be a right arsehole at times, and I'm dejected that I didn't like Dave or take the time to get to know him. With me being... well, the way that I am... let's just say there was no love lost between us. However, Dave didn't let the feelings he must have had for me get in the way of what he did. And bless him for it...

"We were dropping oil, Tony and me, and travelling probably a-hundred-and-forty miles per hour, the both of us, when Dave tried to warn us. He didn't give up, neither, and risked his own life to pull alongside and wave us down. And because of that, when our engine did seize, we were slowing and doing maybe half speed...

"The simple fact of the matter is, if it wasn't for Dave, I wouldn't be breathing right now, and neither would my teammate Tony Dearie. There's not much more I can say, other than this whole experience has taught me a great deal. It's made me a humbler man, I can tell you that for certain, and when I heard this award was going to Dave and Monty, I genuinely couldn't think of anyone more deserving than them and that's the honest truth...

"They have my eternal gratitude and respect."

A standing ovation was given, as Harry McMullan hobbled down from the stage and made his way back to take his place among the other riders.

"Ladies and gentlemen," said Chris, back at the mic. "I'd like to bring his Excellency, the Lieutenant Governor, on stage to present this year's award. And to accept the award on behalf of Dave and Shaun, we're pleased to have Shaun's wife, Tracey, and Dave's brother, Brian, with us."

As the Governor took to the stage, a picture of Dave and Monty appeared, projected up on the screen behind him.

"Bloody hell," said Stan, taking a handkerchief from his tuxedo pocket. "I was doing well, right up until they showed that picture."

"They are a bit difficult on the eyes, aren't they?" said Frank.

Stan laughed, and wiped away the snot bubble that came out his nose.

Frank put a reassuring hand on his knee. "That was a lovely speech by Harry McMullan, though."

"It was indeed," Stan said, in perfect agreement.

"Ladies and Gentlemen," said the Governor. "I've never had the pleasure of meeting them, but, from what I've heard this evening, they sound like delightful lads. It gives me enormous pleasure, then, to present the Spirit of TT Award to David Quirk and Shaun Montgomery."

Monty's wife, Tracey, and Dave's brother, Brian, graciously accepted the award, said a few words, and were on their way again.

"Oh, here I go again," said Stan, taking up his handkerchief once again, to wipe the tears that were now flowing as freely as... well, as tears that flow quite freely.

Chris Kinley took to the stage once more, joining in the applause the audience bestowed upon the award recipients as he did so. "Ladies and gentlemen, two very deserving winners, I'm sure you'll agree."

Giving the lighting technician a nod, the image of Dave and Monty then disappeared.

"And now, by virtue of modern technology, along with permission from the doctors, I'm very pleased to give you, once again... David Quirk and Shaun 'Monty' Montgomery! With sound!"

The screen kicked into life a second time, illuminating the stage. There Dave and Monty were, appearing from their hospital ward with their legs and arms in plaster cast like a scene from a Benny Hill sketch.

"Hello? Is this on?" Dave said, tapping the microphone he'd been given, as if tapping it could suddenly bring it to life if it were not.

"Right. On behalf of Monty and myself, I'd like to say I certainly hope we've passed the audition, and..."

Dave waited for the laughs to come, but the audio was only one-way at the moment.

He tapped the mic again, waggling it around to make sure it was working properly.

"But seriously. I'd like to thank you for this award. It does mean a lot. I've been listening to the award ceremony, and I'd like to say to Harry McMullan to not feel too bad about not liking me, because me and Monty, quite honestly, thought you were a complete dickhead!"

Dave mugged for the camera, waiting again for the laughs. He tapped the microphone yet again, shrugged his shoulders, and carried on.

"Like you, however, we forgive and forget, and we actually like the guy now. In fact, he's bloody brilliant. He's spent hours making us these wheelchairs, which are attached together so we can race around the hospital ward like a sidecar rig! We've yet to try it out, but I'm sure the hospital staff will have loads of fun chasing after us, and a splendid time is guaranteed for all...

"Now's also probably a good time, Harry, to admit that it was us who put the half-pound of salmon in your leathers when you weren't looking, but that's all in the past so no harm done!...

"We'd like to thank you all for this award, and, with your support, we're looking forward to coming back all mended, and better and stronger, next year. Thank you and God bless!"

"I bloody love them two," said Stan, waving at the screen as if they could actually see him. "Oh, and what did they say when you told them, by the way?"

"About what?" asked Frank.

"About Henk offering them a sidecar for next year, one that can really compete?"

"You know Dave," said Frank. "He was too busy looking at the dirty magazines his brother had brought him up."

"He must have said something?" said Stan.

"He did," said Frank. "As his arms were in a cast he asked me to turn the pages!"

"It could've been worse," Stan reminded him. "What with his hands not free and him looking at that sort of magazine and all..."

"Say no more," said Frank. "Stan, we'll be back next year, with Dave and Monty and our charity emblazoned all over the new-and-improved Outfit Number Forty-Two, and you never know, next year we might see him get to a-hundred-and-ten miles per hour."

"I'll drink to that, Frank," said Stan, raising his champagne flute. "And here's to good health!"

"Good health!" said Frank. "And good friends!"

the end

I hope you enjoyed this book. If you did, you may also like the *Lonely Heart Attack Club* series – also based in the Isle of Man.

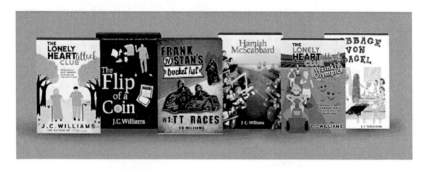

J C Williams
Author

authorjcwilliams@gmail.com
🐦 @jcwilliamsbooks
📘 @jcwilliamsauthor

And check out my latest book,
The Seaside Detective Agency!

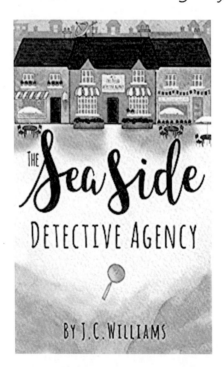